I0145844

Rheumatoid Arthritis

The Best Remedy Guide for Rheumatoid
Arthritis

*(A Guide to the Natural Approach Against
Rheumatoid Arthritis)*

Judith Carrillo

Published By **Phil Dawson**

Judith Carrillo

All Rights Reserved

Rheumatoid Arthritis: The Best Remedy Guide for Rheumatoid Arthritis (A Guide to the Natural Approach Against Rheumatoid Arthritis)

ISBN 978-1-77485-466-2

All rights reserved. No part of this guide may be reproduced in any form without permission in writing from the publisher except in the case of brief quotations embodied in critical articles or reviews.

Legal & Disclaimer

The information contained in this book is not designed to replace or take the place of any form of medicine or professional medical advice. The information in this book has been provided for educational and entertainment purposes only.

The information contained in this book has been compiled from sources deemed reliable, and it is accurate to the best of the Author's knowledge; however, the Author cannot guarantee its accuracy and validity and cannot be held liable for any errors or omissions. Changes are periodically made to this book. You must consult your doctor or get professional medical advice before using any of the suggested remedies, techniques, or information in this book.

Upon using the information contained in this book, you agree to hold harmless the Author from and against any damages, costs, and expenses, including any legal fees potentially resulting from the application of any of the information provided by this guide. This disclaimer applies to any damages or injury caused by the use and application, whether directly or indirectly, of any advice or information presented, whether for breach of contract, tort, negligence, personal injury, criminal intent, or under any other cause of action.

You agree to accept all risks of using the information presented inside this book. You need to consult a professional medical practitioner in order to ensure you are both able and healthy enough to participate in this program.

TABLE OF CONTENTS

Introduction

This book provides the most effective steps and strategies for how to heal arthritis for good once and forever. There are other options too. The description of the disease and all aspects of it are also included to provide more light on the devastating and debilitating illness that has affected fifty million Americans in the current time.

The book explores the autoimmune aspects of arthritis, and delves into the way this immune system can be controlled. The book gives a comprehensive analysis of the current treatments and cures and discusses their pros and cons, benefits and drawbacks, and the newest treatment that is based around immunomodulation.

Thank you so much for purchasing this book. I hope you enjoy it!

Chapter 1: What Is Arthritis?

The phrase "arthritis" can be used quite loosely, and most people refer to it as any type of joint pain or inflammation. If people over an older age complain of stiff or painful joints, we assume that the person suffers from arthritis.

Research in medical and scientific science has revealed that there are more than 100 different forms of arthritis. One author calls it not a single disease, but an amalgamation of ailments with the same characteristics that include joint pain stiffness, inflammation and stiffness. For many people arthritis can limit their ability to walk or standing up, and even writing. If the arthritis is severe the condition may turn into complete degeneration of the joint's protective coating that causes brittle bones, and limit mobility in significant ways. The joints also appear to be damaged. [1]

To differentiate arthritis from other types osteoarthritis (OA) is the most frequent type of arthritis. In the age group of 45 and under there are more males than females who have been diagnosed OA and it is usually caused through physical or bodily injuries and accidents. At the age of 45 the course of the disease shifts: more women than men are identified with OA. 2 Osteoarthritis is extensively discussed in Chapter Four.

The second most common form of arthritis is rheumatoid (RA) which is an inflammatory disease where the body fights against the healthy tissue of its body. Around 3-4 percent in the American population is affected by the condition, and it can be a problem for children. The prevalence of women by RA 3 times as frequently than men. Women who are older than 30 are more likely to be at chance of getting RA People who are born carrying the gene marker HLA-DR4 are also at risk for having higher chances of developing RA. [3]

Other types of arthritis include gout and it is a problem that affects 2 million Americans (in this instance the majority of men are affected than women).

There are other less well-known types of arthritis like ankylosing Spondylitis, the psoriatic arthritis and the infectious arthritis. [4]

With more than 100 kinds that it is now an broad term that covers a range that includes more than 100 ailments which affect nearly 4.3 million Americans. Certain forms of arthritis are affecting infants, while certain forms only manifest at an age.

The over 100 types of arthritis - each having distinctive characteristics - share a commonality They all affect the skeletal and muscular systems and, specifically, in joints, where bones of different sizes meet. A thorough understanding of the joint can assist us in understanding the nature of the disease however, it is mistaken to think that arthritis is limited to joint issues. There are many forms associated with arthritis known as systemic. This means that they may be affecting other parts of the body. They could cause damage to any organ in the body, such as the lungs, the heart kidneys, blood vessels and the skin. [5]

Arthritis is one of the most significant factors that cause disability throughout the United States and accounts for annual medical expenses for in the United States of almost $65 billion.

Be assured that there isn't a lot of doom and doom and. While the number of arthritis cases rises each year, more of arthritis sufferers have a better way of managing their lives due to a mix of natural and medical treatment techniques.

Before we continue our discussion of arthritis, let's talk about the joint since this is the part of the body which is the most affected area when arthritis hits.

Understanding the Joint

A joint is what lets us move in many ways. It's the bridge connecting the 206 bones in our bodies. There are at most three types of joints:

* Hinge joints are knees and elbows, they swing around like the door that opens and closes

* Joints with sockets and ball such as the shoulder or· hip are examples. They allow people to pivot

and turn in a variety of directions, while remaining connected to one another.

Other kinds of joints include those on the pelvis which move small amount, and others that remain completely solid and don't move in any way. Some examples are the joints inside the skull.

In spite of this wide the range of motion joints aren't without limits. They are able to function well when they are they are regularly used, however when they are used in overuse, they may be damaged.

A number of bones join to create an joint. The human body is home to around 150 "linkages." These bones' ends are covered by a soft tissue called cartilage. It absorbs shocks and allows joints to function without a hitch. Certain joints are equipped with small, bursae, which are filled with fluid. The joint is encased within a capsule comprised of connective tissue and is lined with a fine membrane known as the synovium. The synovium's exit is a synovial fluid, which helps to lubricate joints and aiding in movement. [6]

Soft tissues, in addition to muscles, support and surround the joints. Muscles are made up of flexible fibers which help move areas within the human body. Tendons are the muscles' fibers in the end of muscles, and connect them with bones. Ligaments are supportive tissues which are linked to bones and hold them together in a joint.

Any or all of the structures mentioned above could be affected by any of the types of arthritis.

If you feel in pain or is "disjointed" or "disjointed," it is essential to see a physician who can identify the issue since it is crucial to determine the type of arthritis is present prior to deciding on the medication or treatment suggested. The main question isn't "do you have arthritis?" but "what kind of arthritis do I suffer from?"

With an understanding of the basics of the joint, we'll look at the "faces" of arthritis, as defined by the Mayo Clinic. It's been a mystery on the cause of arthritis, as per the Mayo Clinic, but the human effects of arthritis are very obvious. The cause could result from genetic influences (such as the cases of rheumatoid and many other types) or injuries or other types or physical injury (as as in osteoarthritis).

Other reasons could be absence of physical activity as well as aging processes, excess weight, an imbalanced immune system, the influence of your environment (food as well as water sources) as well as an imbalance in the enzymes. Stress can cause symptoms to worsen. It is suggested that stress can make symptoms worse. Mayo Clinic enumerates the following symptoms that are related to arthritis and its various forms: [77. (note that the two most prevalent forms of arthritis - osteoarthritis as well as Rheumatoid Arthritis - can be abbreviated to OA as well as RA in both cases).

* Cartilage breakdown is a common occurrence when there is OA or RA,

Inflammation of the synovial membrane and muscles, blood vessels, ligaments, and tendons. It occurs in arthritis that is inflammatory.

* The formation of crystals within the synovial fluid, which can cause acute gout as well as pseudogout.

* Shrinkage or shrinkage of tendons or muscles leading to joint deformities - is a common occurrence in all types of arthritis when the joint is immobile,

* Skin tightening is a common occurrence in scleroderma.

* Organ damage that is internal may occur as a result of RA and other types of inflammatory arthritis.

* Inability to move joints can occur as the result of joint injury or weak muscles

The muscle's strength is reduced - occurs when a joint is not being used for a long periodof time,

* Reduced mobility occurs due to the long-term absence exercising or joint injuries and may last for a long time.

Chapter 2: Rheumatoid Adhritis

What exactly is Rheumatoid Arthritis?

This must be made explicit from the beginning that Rheumatoid arthritis (RA) is distinct than osteoarthritis (OA). RA is a condition that affects the immune system of the body.

While OA can affect cartilage and causes its destruction, RA is even more grave. It's like the human body's attempt to fight foreign invaders. In the same way, RA destroys or damages the joints via an immune system. The synovium has been inflamed. the thin membrane that surrounds the joints.

There are around 2.5 million Americans suffering from RA. Contrary to OA that can cause destruction slowly, the harm that is caused by RA can be accelerated in way. In just a few months or even years, people suffering of RA might have joints that are deformed which cause a lot of discomfort, however, their other organs can be affected, leading to symptoms of fatigue and fever and issues with the skin or blood vessels, lung or even heart. [1]

The joints of people who suffer of RA can be affected in asymmetrical manner this means that the moment one knee or elbow is painful and inflamed and painful, the opposite knee or elbow will also be painful and inflamed. The joints most often damaged by RA are fingers, hands wrists, elbows, ankles, knees, shoulders and feet.

It was mentioned previously that an individual's immune system is attacking healthy tissues is at fault however, doctors aren't exactly what causes this. One possible explanation is that it's a result of environmental and genetic factors HLA-DR4, a gene markers, is discovered as a factor in the process of developing RA.

The environmental causes, such as bacteria or viral infections as well as cigarette smoke and coffee are also associated with RA. Women who smoke older have three times the chance of developing RA higher than women who do not smoke. A study from Finland found that people who drank more than four cups of caffeine were two times more likely develop the rheumatoid-related factor which is an antibody that can cause RA. [2]

Furthermore, as RA is more prevalent in females than males, one causes has been linked with hormonal changes.

The signs and symptoms of Rheumatoid Arthritis

Stiffness, pain, swelling as well as loss of joint function are the main symptoms of RA. The condition affects the finger and wrist joints that are closest in proximity to hand however, as previously mentioned, it can be affecting other areas other than joints. Patients with RA might experience extreme fatigue as well as fevers, and an overall feeling of being unwell.

It is reported that the National Institutes of Health (NIH) stated that RA can last from between a few months and an entire year for certain individuals but without causing significant or lasting damage, however, others might experience just mild or moderate symptoms and may experience periods where these symptoms get more severe or experience flare-ups.

The symptoms sufferers of RA:

* Swollen joints. Joints feel warm and tender to the touch.

The affected joints exhibit the same pattern of symmetry,

* Joint inflammation can also lead to swelling and inflammation in the shoulders, neck the elbows, hips, ankles, knees, and feet.

* Fever, fatigue, and occasional generally feeling of being unwell.

Feeling well,

* Soreness and pain lasting longer than 30 minutes in the morning , or following long periods of time of rest. [3]

RA symptoms can be present for many years The RA symptoms can last for a long time, and there is no commonality of symptoms between those suffering from RA. Some people may experience better health - this happens when they're in Remission. The less fortunate suffer from chronic symptoms that persist and can last for a long time. This is the time when RA results in arthritis and causes disability, which deprives their mobility and the living quality.

One of the characteristics that is characteristic of RA has been that it can affect other body parts. Patients suffering from RA can develop anemia or the condition can reduce the production of red blood cells. Dry eyes, neck pain and mouth are other typical symptoms. While it's not often, RA can also inflame blood vessels in an individual's body as well as the lining of lung or the sac that surrounds the heart. [4]

What causes Rheumatoid Arthritis?

The field of RA continues to be a puzzle for medical professionals and the need to research is more fervent than ever. It is difficult to determine the exact cause of RA or even what theories have been developed. One theory is that it's genetic.

Genetics

Scientists have long been of the belief that genetics play a major role in determining whether family members are also susceptible to the illness. It has been suggested the moment one family member suffers from RA the other family member is between three and four times more likely to get RA.

Genetics is a significant factor as children get half their genetic material from their dad while the remaining half comes from their mother.

The significance of genes was in studies of twins. According to Koehn and colleagues If twins are identical in the event that one develops RA in one, then it's likely that the other twin will also develop RA. Because identical twins have genetically identical genes and have the same genetic makeup, it is likely that both will be diagnosed with RA. In the event of identical twins, the possibilities of one developing RA are lower.

This particular genetic component leads humans to the antigen human leucocyte (HLA). This substance plays a crucial function in the ability of humans to either reject or accept kidneys or heart, or any other organ transplanted. The research studies on HLA provide insight into the research into RA and the genetic basis.

It was found that a distinct HLA gene marker known as HLA-DRB1 was identified in more RA cases than normal. It was discovered that the connection to RA was limited to a small portion of the HLADRB1 amino acid proteins that range from between 67 and 74, and the sequence "forms the smallest docking station within the molecules. A high percentage of this docking station can be found in the genes of those suffering from RA."[55

Although this could be regarded as to be a major breakthrough in the study of RA but scientists remain cautious about it due to the fact that it's not the whole story. It is evident that more research needs to be done. One benefit of this research breakthrough is that we are now aware that there are a variety of RA genes. Certain of these genes trigger the disease to begin and the others may be the cause of longevity of the condition.

The link between genetics and RA is a complex matter This is the reason why the heart research of RA research is the research of RA genes. To discover the genes that are that are unique for RA, American scientists are working in tandem with researchers from around the globe to gather data on 1000 families where at least one member suffers from RA. The new techniques that weren't utilized before aren't being developed to the point that the identification of RA genes becomes a simpler task.

Scientists are discovering something new about RA every day. Every bit of wisdom gathered is used to develop effective treatments to RA sufferers.

Abnormal Bowel Permeability

It is a condition that is common in those with RA which is characterized by an increase in intestinal permeability. There is a belief that foods sensitivities are a major factor in increasing the risk of intestinal permeability during rheumatoid arthritis.

If a person has a leaky stomach and is susceptible to absorbing massive amounts of dietary and bacterial molecules increases. Because the molecules are too large they are prevented from being absorbed. However, for those suffering from RA the molecules are absorbed from the body. The body then produces antibodies to bind to them. When immune cells release antibodies they are able to attach to foreign molecules such as those that are found on viruses, bacteria and cancerous cells. This leads to the creation the immune system. [6]

It might sound unfamiliar to some readers however, we are now getting to the idea of cross-reacting antibodies. These antibodies are your body's method of generating antibodies against the tissue it is in. When intestinal permeability is raised while the intestinal flora altered this means that the antigens that are taken in are the same as those that are found in the joints' tissues. [7]

In RA it's the molecules in bacteria and food that act as antigens which are bound by antibodies. Your body's immune system releases chemicals to destroy the immune system. When these substances settle in joints they do not just destroy the immune system, but also the surrounding tissue. [8]

Researchers have discovered there is a key contributor to the growth of RA that causes the development of inflammation and damage. When joint tissues are destroyed the large molecules are exposed because they're not covered by the cell membrane or connective tissue.

Patients with RA thus have symptoms of a change in the bacteria flora as well as a small intestinal overgrowth. This imbalance is related to the severity of the symptoms and the severity of disease. [9]

The explanation is simplified way through Dr. Braly, Medical Director of Immuno Labs of Florida, RA is a condition in which the body fights against its own tissues. The most common cause of illness is delayed food allergy, which is the issue of an abnormal permeability in the wall of your intestinal as the Dr. Braly said.

Based on the research of Dr. Braly, food particles which haven't been fully eliminated (owing to this permeability issue) traverse the digestive tract before getting to the bloodstream. If they're not cleared by the body, they end up being deposited within tissues which can then trigger an inflammation reaction. Also, since our bodies are allergic food particles that have been deposited the result is an autoimmune condition which causes tissue damage surrounding joints. [11]

Other causes of Rheumatoid Arthritis

Although genetics play an important part in RA however, there are many other elements that contribute to the condition.

One reason that is often mentioned is the environment. While a bacterial or viral disease can cause RA Scientists aren't able to determine what the specific agent is. It is imperative to keep in mind however it is important to remember that RA is not transmissible. It isn't transferable between people. the next.

Other reasons may be due to hormonal causes. RA is more often diagnosed for women. Pregnancy can make the disease worse however it may be triggered after pregnancy. [12]

Breastfeeding can also worsen the symptoms. Birth control medications can reduce the likelihood of becoming afflicted with RA. Researchers believe that the levels of immune system substances interleukin 12 (IL-12) and tumor necrosis factor alpha (TNF-a) could change with changes in hormone levels. This could cause the tissue damage and swelling that is seen in RA.

Certain hormonal deficiencies or hormones can trigger the formation of RA for a person who is genetically susceptible , and who might have been exposed to a trigger environmental trigger.

Although the reasons behind it are not understood but there is a certain assertion that could be madethat says RA results through the interaction of various elements. Research is ongoing to discover these causes and their interactions. [13]

Chapter 3: Natural Treatments To Arthritis

Researchers and doctors who specialize in studying arthritis often declare that food and arthritis create a bizarre couple.

There isn't any definitive information on what the best diet for those suffering from arthritis. There are no food or food groups that have been found to specifically shield someone from developing arthritis or help relieve it.

What arthritis experts are aware of is that certain foods which can trigger flare-ups in arthritis for those who are susceptible to flare-ups, and it's in this space that those suffering from arthritis may be active in dealing with their issues. Certain doctors have advised patients to narrow on the foods which trigger flare-ups with careful surveillance, so that once they are discovered, they can be removed completely from their diet.

Food & Diet

Food is a powerful factor that needs to be considered in arthritis. If people consume certain kinds of food, they could trigger pain and swelling symptoms by altering the functions in the body's immune system. Certain patients who work closely together with nutrition advisors have had success in slowly eliminating the foods that trigger arthritic pain.

Before we discuss the benefits of food as a natural treatment for arthritis, we have be aware of the concept that food-related allergies exist. There are three kinds of allergies: fixed as well as cyclic allergies. an addictive allergy.

An allergy that is fixed that is caused by the immune system results in constant and invariable reaction to food, regardless of frequency or frequency. [1]

A cyclic allergy is an allergic reaction which is caused by a decreasing symptoms of the triggering food, provided that enough period of time passes between the initial and second meal which contains the flare-up that is causing the food. The normal cycle time as per the doctor Dr. John Irwin, is between five and seven days because between meals the immune system has the capability of "forgetting" the extent to which it hates the food of the enemy.

Yet, the memory is only partial, since when a person eats on that same day, and the next day the immune system has regrouped, resulting in an arthritis reaction. [2]

Third allergy known as an addictive allergy. It can cause some symptoms when food is consumed by the body. It can trigger more intense reactions when the food is removed. Coffee is a good example. There are people who experience headaches after not drinking coffee for several hours. When they finally do have coffee it is gone.

The issue of allergies leads an end to, by removing food-related allergies, people who suffer from RA may find some kind of relief from their pain and discomfort. If they consume the right kinds of foods and adhering to an appropriate lifestyle patients can lessen their RA symptoms.

Although doctors are unable to pinpoint specific food items that trigger flare-ups in the body, studies have identified the most frequently triggering foods such as corn, wheat milk, dairy products as well as dark-colored foods such as potato, tomato as well as eggplant, peppers, and tobacco. The addition of certain ingredients has also been proven to aggravate arthritis.

A study carried out by the University of Oslo, Norway several years back showed a treatment group as opposed to a group of non-treatment participants who received different diets. The group that was treated followed an energizing diet, fasting for between five and seven days. The food provided to the participants consisted of vegetable broth, garlic and juices of beets, carrots and celery. No fruit juices were allowed.

Following the fasting and after the fasting period, a new food item was introduced every day. If the group experienced increased pain, or feeling stiff or swollen they stopped eating the food for seven days prior to introducing it for the second time. If they experienced the same pain the pain was eliminated automatically.

RA patients are advised to eat fresh fruits vegetables whole grains, whole grains, dairy products that are low in fat and proteins that are lean and low in fat. It is also recommended to eat foods high in flavonoids, bromelain omega-3 fats as well as vitamins C and E as well as zinc.

Drinking green tea , and eating turmeric and ginger could be beneficial. In actual fact, lower rates of RA has been found for those who drink regularly green tea. The catechins present contained in teas like green are thought to reduce cartilage breakdown and reduce chronic joint inflammation.

Below are some foods RA patients should consume regularly to ease discomforts caused by RA discomforts:

Cold Water Fish

Baked halibut is a great way to soothe joint pain. It has been observed that those who consume large portions of fish frequently are at a lower risk of developing RA.

The advantages of omega-3 fat acids can't be denied. Many people suffering from RA have seen improvement in the way they feel. A serving of 4 to 6 servings of fish per week is recommended by medical professionals in order to get the beneficial fats. Examples of cold-water fish are mackerel, salmon, halibut herring, tuna as well as cod, sardines, and cod.

Vitamin D-rich Foods

Tuna, salmon shrimp, salmon and eggs, sunflower seeds as well as vitamin D-fortified milk products are all examples of foods that are high in vitamin D. they provide some protection from the development of RA. The information was published in a Jan. 2004 edition of Arthritis and Rheumatism.

Fruits and vegetables

Vegetables that are cooked, steamed, stir-friedor roasted or grilled are a great addition in any healthy diet program. Fresh vegetables and fruits contain anti-inflammatory antioxidants such as Vitamin C as well as vitamin E. Many are also rich with fiber which help to restore the healthy balance of beneficial bacteria in the gut, thus reducing inflammation throughout the body.

Positive studies show positive results. RA patients who are eating fruits and vegetables have improved or are gone completely. Some have even stopped taking painkillers, but those who are just beginning eating a diet are advised to not discontinue their medications abruptly.

Olive Oil

Countries in the Mediterranean such as Greece, Italy, Sicily and other countries whose food is abundant in vegetables, fruits whole grains, powerful spices, as well as pure extra-virgin olive oil generally have lower rates of RA by up to 75 percent.

Prostacyclin is an extremely powerful anti-inflammatory chemical that is found in the fats of olive oil. Certain RA patients also experience less symptoms once they start the olive oil treatment. [4]

Yogurt

While not proven scientifically drinking a cup of yogurt in place of baking goods as an afternoon snack could ease RA symptoms. The bacteria in the dairy products that are fermented are the same beneficial bacteria that live in the gut, which help protect our bodies from the harmful bacteria. The yogurt you purchase should claims to contain active, live cultures as certain yogurts are heated to kill bacteria prior to being sold. [5]

Supplements (and certain plant-based supplements)

The US Arthritis Foundation in its book, Managing Your Arthritis, has created a whole section on nutritional supplements for RA patients.

The Foundation however, cautions that patients with RA explore a variety of natural remedies, such as adding supplements to their daily diet. Some have experienced significant improvement in their overall health. However, that doesn't mean that they're scientifically validated.

Current trends are moving toward alternative treatments (also called non-proven cures) which is most noticeable among those who live with constant discomfort and are unable to not take the medication, no matter the strength of the doses. If the treatment doesn't work then who is to blame people who wish to try everything?

The majority of the issues are psychological, too. Being convinced that alternative therapy will help can provide relief. It is a good thing for arthritis sufferers, the rising popularity of supplements as well as other treatments have made it necessary for researchers to study the subject more deeply.

The public is not hindered from trying the numerous options as they can however they should follow the advice of their physician. It is important to keep in mind that the so-called natural remedies might not be 100 percent organic. RA patients could also be at risk when they are taking medications with herbal remedies, which can cause adverse reactions.

Nutritional supplements are comprised of herbs, vitamins, animal compounds, and minerals. They are available in all places and are accompanied by promises of immediate relief from ailments.

Let's take a look at some of the supplements arthritis sufferers have been recognized to take:

Glucosamine

This is a highly regarded nutritional supplement, one of the most sought-after supplements particularly for people suffering from osteoarthritis. While it isn't a cure many are reporting feeling more comfortable when their pain lessens and stiffness reduces.

It is extracted by shrimp, crab and lobster shells. There is an idea that it slows the degrading of cartilage. 6. NIH is researching this supplement right now. It is safe, and, if you are able to pay for it the Foundation suggests that individuals take it for a test. But people with diabetes may want to speak with their doctor prior to taking glucosamine. [7]

Chondroitin Sulfate

It is produced by the body and it's believed that it directs fluid to the cartilage in order to make it elastic and more durable. This substance is extracted from the tracheas of cattle, and when combined with glucosamine, it is believed to alleviate the symptoms of osteoarthritis. [8]

No adverse reactions have been documented.

Boswellia

The ingredient is derived directly from the Asian tree and is believed to block leukotriene synthesis, which is a factor in inflammation. However, studies have failed to establish that it can alleviate pain for people suffering from arthritis. The most frequent negative side effects are skin rash, diarrhea nausea, and a rash. However, it is considered to be to be safe.

Cat's Claw

The substance is derived from a tree that grows throughout the Peruvian Amazon It has been used for centuries of relieving bone inflammation and pain. A study conducted on a single animal showed a decrease of pain and inflammation however, no studies have been conducted on human beings. [9]

Celadrin

Celadrin is an anti-inflammatory substance that naturally occurs in the body that is safe for mobility and joint flexibility. It is composed by esterification of fatty acids. It acts on a cell level to ease swelling and inflammation. With time, the usage can reduce the degeneration of cartilage in joints.

It can be found in both oral and topical forms. It is completely safe with minimal or no adverse negative effects that have been reported in studies done on it. It is generally safe to use in conjunction with other prescription drugs however, it is recommended to consult with your physician prior to taking Celadrin.

Chapter 4: Natural Vs Medical Treatment For

Arthritis

The most unfortunate aspect of RA is that those who suffer from it require long-term treatment that consists of physical therapy, medications regularly exercising and education.

The section on medical treatment will cover the use of surgery and medication, after which , a discussion of natural treatments will be discussed.

Medication

(1) The DMARD is typically after the confirmation of RA is established, RA patients are advised to begin a vigorous treatment plan that includes exercising, rest and rest to build bone and muscle and disease-modifying anti-rheumatic medicines also known as DMARDs.

One DMARD most frequently recommended is Methotrexate (Rheumatrex). Other DMARDs include leflunomide (Arava) and the gold thiomalate (Myochrysine) as well as aurothioglucose (Solganal) as well as the auranofin (Ridaura). [1]

(2) NSAIDS - are non-steroidal anti-inflammatory medications which are also given by doctors to RA patients. Examples include ibuprofen (Motrin, Advil) as well as fenoprofen. indomethacin as well as naproxen (Naprosyn).

To alleviate joints and joint inflammation RA sufferers are prescribed NSAIDS. They are very effective, however, prolonged use may result in abdominal issues such as bleeding and ulcers. Certain MSAIDS are also recognized to cause heart issues. They US Food and Drug Administration has ordered drug makers of NSAIDs to alert consumers of a higher risk of heart problems and digestive bleeding. [2]

(3) COX-2 inhibitors these kinds of drugs are designed to inhibit COX-2 which is an enzyme that causes inflammation. They function as effectively as NSAIDs however they cause less stomach discomfort. The US FDA however, is currently investigating several reports of COX-2 causing strokes and heart attacks. Two COX-2 drugs have

been removed from the marketplace: Rofecoxib (Vioxx) and valdecoxib (Bextra).

An additional COX-2 inhibitor called Celecoxib (Celebrex) is in stock, however, when it is offered to the general public is accompanied by an advisory. Patients are advised to get the lowest dose that can be used in the shortest time. Patients should ask their doctors regarding whether the COX-2 medicine is suitable and safe for them.

(4) Antimalarial drugs (the NIH states that antimalarial drugs like the hydroxychloroquine (Plaquenil) and Sulfasalazine (Azulfidine) are useful, and typically used in conjunction with DMARD methotrexate. Patients must wait for some time before experiencing any of the benefits of these medicines. Patients given these drugs are required to have regular blood tests due to the toxic effects they can cause. [3]

(5) Tumor necrosis factor (TNF) inhibitors are new classes of drugs to treat an autoimmune disorder. These comprise Etanercept (Enbrel) as well as infliximab (Remicade) and the adalimumab (Humira). Adalimumab and

etanercept can be injected medicines. Infliximab can be administered via infusion. [4]

(6) Kineret It is also a drug that is new and is referred to as an injectable anakinra Brand name: Kineret. It is a human-made protein that can be used to block interleukin-1, an inflammation-related protein. Kineret can slow the progression of severe and moderate RA for patients aged 18 or older who haven't had a favorable response to DMARDs and TNF inhibitors.

(7) Corticosteroids - these drugs are designed to decrease RA inflammation. They may cause adverse consequences, which is why they are only prescribed for short-term use as well as at lower doses when appropriate. Corticosteroids users may be afflicted with psychosis, bruising weight gain, cataracts vulnerability to diabetes, infections as well as high blood pressure and bone thinning (osteoporosis). [5]

Surgery

Since RA can result in severe disfigured joints, surgery may assist in relieving joint discomfort, eliminate deformities and improve the functioning of joints, but only to a small extent.

The knees and the hips are the two areas where the most successful surgeries are carried out. Sysnovectomy is usually the first procedure and involves elimination of the membrane that surrounds the joint, namely synovium.

Another alternative procedure could include the replacement of an entire joint using prosthesis. The NIH states that in extreme instances, total hip or knee replacement could make a huge different between complete dependence on others and autonomy at home.

Natural Treatment

The major distinction between natural and medical remedies for RA is pretty obvious : the presence or non-existence of any medication. As we mentioned previously, medical treatment could be surgical or medication or both based on severity symptoms.

Natural remedies would tend toward implementing lifestyle and diet adjustments and a controlled fitness program, with regular intakes of herbal or natural supplements.

Concerning the use of natural remedies for RA and RA, we look toward Doctor. Weil, that famous doctor who has a beard that is a regular on TV and has gained a huge fan base due to his straightforward method of treating any illness. He also advocates of alternative treatments that are natural and advises RA patients against NSAIDs and DMARDs due to their long-term effects. He also states that those who depend on these medications tend to not be responsive to natural therapies.

Here are a few examples of Dr. Weil's most fundamental strategies for dealing with RA:

(1) Maintain an extremely low-protein, high-carbohydrate diet The doctor. Weil advises RA sufferers to limit their intake of food products derived from animals.

(2) Eliminate dairy products and milk in your diet daily,

(3) Avoid margarine vegetable oils, and all products that contain partially hydrogenated oils

(4) Enhance the omega-3 fatty acids in your regular meals by eating more chilled waters,

flaxseeds, or walnuts. Supplementing with fish oil can also aid.

(5) Participate in an aerobics program with Doctor. Weil recommends swimming particularly for RA patients.

(6) Develop relaxation methods. Adding visualization is also helpful in reducing the autoimmune response, and psychotherapy may help to change emotions that can cause an imbalance in our immune system. Hypnotherapy as well as guided imagery are suggested.

(7) Yoga and meditation have proved "their power" as they say and RA sufferers might discover that these methods of healing can help alleviate symptoms.

(8) Remove smoking and coffee from your diet as both are known for increasing risk of RA.

The good thing concerning RA can be that it might allow patients enter Remission within their first year. About 20% of patients suffer from remission in the 10-to-15 years after the first diagnosis.

Over half (50 70 to 80 percent) of those who are able to have an employment full-time.

After about 15-20 years 10% of patients develop severe disabilities and are unable to perform their normal activities. [7]

Chapter 5: Osteoarthritis

What exactly is Osteoarthritis?

A Englishman, John Kent Spender (1829-1916) was mentioned by The British Medical Journal as saying, "Few things are so likely to induce a state of dismay at a medical gathering because of the possibility of a discussion on...osteoarthritis. This field seems so barrenthat the harvest is insignificant. ..."[1[]

That was in 1888. It is doubtful that the field is today, but the harvest is definitely quite large.

Research into osteoarthritis has made great strides!

Osteoarthritis is among the most frequent of the rheumatic diseases that are that are recognized through the Arthritis Foundation of the US. It is described as a degenerative condition of joints. More specifically, it's a form of arthritis that attacks cartilage articular in the joint. [2]

The articular cartilage acts as an enveloping sponge that covers the bones' ends once they come into contact with the joint. A good example is the femur (bone located in the upper thigh) as well as the tibia (shin bone) coming together in the knee. The articular cartilage is thought to function to act as shock absorption, or as a cushion within the joint. Because it's a slippery material that allows joints to move between each other smoothly.

Osteoarthritis occurs when the articular cartilage starts to wear and tear and cannot function effectively. As it deteriorates, it shrinks and becomes less dense. Without this cartilage bones suffer from injury and start to get caught in the cross-fire. [3]

Signs and symptoms of Osteoarthritis

The most prominent signs of osteoarthritis based on the joint affected, are:

* Pain

* Stiffness

* Bony swelling and enlargement

Patients suffering from severe osteoarthritis may be unable to perform the most basic of tasks like opening jars or climbing steps getting more difficult as joints experience progressive decline. The majority of cases of osteoarthritis are concentrated on a couple of joints initially and they're typically the joints that bear weight, such as the knee, hip or spine, hands, and hand joints that are small.

Let's start with the first indication that is discomfort (accompanied by a diminished movement).

Osteoarthritis pain can be due to injury in the joint. Pain is experienced in or around the joint affected and patients experience a restricted mobility. The pain gets worse with time and people experience the most pain during the early mornings.

The reason why patients experience joint pain is due to the growth of bone that occur when they touch.

The patients with osteoarthritis also experience discomfort when they bend, kneel or climb steps. As the cartilage thins away, the cushioning that cushions bones decreases. The pain can be very severe, especially when the cartilage has gone through a decline, which causes the joint to become unstable.

It is interesting to note that osteoarthritis may cause the doctors refer to as "referred discomfort." It is a type of discomfort that is not present in the joint affected but is felt in different areas, such as the buttocks or groin region, knee, or thigh. [5]

As expected it is expected that a spinal arthritis can cause pain that spreads into the arms, neck or legs. Osteoarthritis pain may also be more severe following a stressful time in life, such as a loss of job or divorce.

Stiffness is a second sign of osteoarthritis. The stiffness can be felt following some time of inactivity, when you are sitting or sleeping for a long time. The stiffness could last for up to 30 minutes, and then slowly diminishes as the person starts to move around as the joint is warmed up.

The third sign is swelling and bony enlargement. When cartilage begins to break down it is possible for bony growths to expand or spurs develop. These are the spurs are visible in the swollen and achy appearance of people suffering from osteoarthritis.

Causes for Osteoarthritis (OA)

Michael Murray, ND says Michael Murray, ND says that OA is classified into two types Primary and Secondary.

In primary OA the wear that happens with age manifests itself as stiffness and joint pain - typically around 50 or 60 years old. Primary OA is not a predicate of a prior injury. As we age, our system's ability to repair and create cartilage structures diminishes. Repair of important enzymes is also significantly reduced. Primarily OA is therefore a result of age, more so than any other condition.

Secondary OA is associated with an underlying factor such as inherited issues with joint function or structure trauma, the presence of abnormal cartilage, and previous joint inflammation disorder, like RA or Gout. [7]

The Natural Ways to Treat OA

Food

The majority of physicians believe that diet plays an important part in the treatment and prevention of OA. A healthy diet is essential to achieve the main objective of therapy which is to improve the joint repair mechanisms.

The most important factor to consider is whether the diet consumed by the OA patient is abundant in vegetables and fruits. The cells of our bodies are always being attacked by free radicals, which results in diseases like OA and also heart disease, cancer or Alzheimer's disease, as well as any other chronic degenerative diseases. Even though the body is trying to make free radicals surrounding environment can significantly increase a person's burden of free radicals. Smoking tobacco is one example of how it can cause the depletion of antioxidants such for Vitamin C as well as beta-carotene.

Dr. Murray believes that antioxidants and human enzymes found in food sources can help protect us from the harm caused from free radicals. Food ingredients that are able to protect people are flavonoids, carotenes Vitamins C & E, as well as sulfur-containing compounds. Consuming a variety of these compounds in fresh vegetables and fruits can boost the concentrations of these tissues. Patients suffering from OA or any other type of arthritis are advised to drink fresh juices of fruits and vegetables The best device to have at hand is the juicer. [9]

Some of the most beneficial food options to treat OA mentioned by Murray suggests to patients. Murray mentions are:

* Blueberries, cherries, and blackberries

* Garlic onions, garlic, Brussel sprouts, and cabbage

Supplements for Nutrition

In addition to a balanced diet, supplements to aid in nutrition can be a great aid for people who suffer from OA. The body needs antioxidants such as manganese, selenium as well as Vitamins C & E is vital as are the nutrients responsible for the creation of certain joint-specific substances including niacinamide and pantothenic acid, Vitamin B6 and zinc are especially important.

(1) The primary natural substance Dr. Murray points to is it's glucosamine, which is the same substance that is recommended by doctors for RA patients. Dr. Murray claims that it is "nature's most effective treatment for OA...because it's primary purpose is to increase the production of cartilage-related components." Thus the glucosamine ingredient is an important component in joint rehabilitation.

In double-blind studies, the glucosamine has been found to give more effective results than other NSAIDs or placebos. Dr. Murray's opinion that NSAIDs are designed to relieve symptoms, but could actually contribute to the progress of the disease while glucosamine targets the source of the problem. It addresses the root of OA. It does not just relieve pain, but it also assists the body to repair damaged joints. [10]

In terms of adverse effects are concerned, glucosamine does not cause any adverse effects and is totally safe, unlike NSAIDs. The benefits of glucosamine are evident when used for a long time. Given that it's not a painkiller or an anti-inflammatory drug, it does not show results right away. However, over time the effects felt by certain OA patients are astonishing.

Glucosamine can be found in many health food stores as well as in supermarkets. But, it is recommended to purchase the sulfate in lieu of N-acetyglucosamine or glucosamine hydrochloride. [11]

(2) Vitamins C & E are both good antioxidants that can help reduce the damage to cartilage. If there is no Vitamin C in joint tissues the collagen synthesis ceases. Insufficient Vitamin C concentrations are typical among people who are elderly. There are studies in the lab that suggest that the greater the amount of Vitamin C is, the higher the chance of protection against OA.

Dr. Murray shares Dr. Linus Pauling's belief that during situations of illness or stress people must boost the amount of Vitamin C and they must supplement their diets by consuming between 1,000 and three milligrams Vitamin C every day. OA patients should be able to find other food sources for Vitamin C from food items.

Vitamin E is, on contrary is known to have certain membrane stabilizing properties as well as preventing the destruction of cartilage. It also aids in the creation of cartilage elements. Certain experts have suggested using Vitamins C & E together.

(3) Niacinamide - a type that is a form of Vitamin B3. One famous doctor named Dr. Kaufman, was said to have helped thousands of OA sufferers using niacinamide, which is a substance that is much more well-tolerated than Niacin. One word of caution not to take too much Niacinamide can cause damage to the liver It is therefore recommended to take this supplement under an expert's guidance, especially when you exceed 9,000 mg is consumed daily. Tests for liver function each three-month period are suggested.

(4) 4. Pantothenic acid is one of the forms of Vitamin B5 which is an essential ingredient to promote cartilage growth. The Dr. Murray, however, warns that , while small doses of this substance every day may bring some benefit to OA patients, greater doses haven't seen significant improvements.

(5) Vitamins B6, A, and E. Zinc, Baron and Copper All of them are vital to maintain normal cartilage and collagen. A healthy intake can be obtained by taking a high-quality multi-vitamin or multi mineral formula which provides an RDA for these minerals. Boron is a bit different and can be obtained from vegetables and fruits. Germany has been using boron supplements to treat OA in the late 70's due to the role it plays in treating OA.

Plant-based medicines

Nutritional and botanical agents are often recommended for inflammation. Plant extracts that are beneficial include curcumin (a ingredient in the spice tumeric) as well as ginger.

Plants that are rich in compounds called phytoestrogens are often employed. They are able to bind with receptors for estrogen on cartilage cells. Due to the increased frequency of OA among women, estrogens may have a role to play. Some of the botanicals that are utilized to combat OA include licorice root dong quai and alfalfa. [12]

One method of increasing the amount of phytoestrogens in your diet is to eat food items that are rich in them. Sources of food include:

* Fennel

* Celery

* Parsley

* Soy

* Nuts

* Whole grains

* Apples

Consuming these food items along with alfalfa and licorice tea sprouts is more beneficial rather than taking small doses of herb. Women in menopausal stages are strongly encouraged to consume phytoestrogen-rich herbs.

Boswellia The full term refers to Boswellia serrata, which is a massive tree that is native to India. Boswellic acids have been shown to have anti-arthritic properties in a variety of animal studies. Furthermore, clinical trials involving humans have produced positive results in both OA as well as RA. The recommended dose is around 400 mg three times a day. There have been no side effects identified. [13]

Devil's Claw - this plant is believed to have a long history of being used to treat arthritis. It is believed to have an anti-inflammatory analgesic properties that are comparable to those of phenylbutazone which is a potent medication. However, clinical studies have not proved its effectiveness 100.

Doctor. Murray believes that devil's claw may be better at treating gout. He suggests this dose three times a day:

Dried powdered root 1 - 2 grams or in tea

Tincture from 4 -6 milliliters (1 to 1 teaspoon)

Dry extracts of solids 400 mg

Training and physical therapy

There are many exercises OA patients can take part in We will give an overview of the exercises that patients can do. OA patients are advised to consult their doctors and physical therapists regarding the possibility of a fitness program. While exercise is proven to be beneficial to OA patients, certain exercises can be detrimental. A close supervision is essential.

The most important element of any fitness program is warming up and stretching.

Regular stretching is important for everyone, whether Olympic participants, arthritis sufferers or those who simply are looking to maintain their fitness. Most people do not stretch enough, yet it's an essential component of any fitness program because it helps keep the body supple and flexible. It also prepares muscles for fitness routine, whether aerobic or weight lifting.

When stretching in stretching, steady and slow moves are recommended.

Be sure to follow these rules of thumb:

* Warm up prior to stretching,

Relax as you move into an exercise, take a moment to relax while you're in the stretch , and ease off your tension. Take deep and consistent breaths.

Don't bounce when stretching.

* Relax into a Stretch until there is some tension. If you experience discomfort, you've stretched too much.

Concentrate on your the form while stretching. This results in greater flexibility as you get stronger,

Keep in mind that flexibility does not last forever. There will be occasions when you're feeling like your body isn't as flexible and "long" as it is on other instances. Stretch comfortably and do not force yourself to stretch. You'll regain your old flexibility with time.

If you experience a feeling of weakness or illness when stretching, stop and tell your physician as it could be an indication of a heart problem.

Before starting an exercise program it is recommended to discuss the following aspects with your doctor or physical therapist

* Fitness level

* Age

* Preference to exercise alone or in groups

* Preference for where to exercise

* Budgetary considerations

* Time limitations

* Preference for one or more sport

Each of these variables affect the way in which your trainer or doctor will determine the best workout program. It will also affect your desire to follow a specific program. Many people get frustrated because they get bored quickly or do not have time, or they want to stay away from injury and discomfort.

It is also important to exercise often. 20 minutes of exercise per day is enough. Thirty minutes is better. [15]

The types of exercises for OA patients are able to perform could be any combination one or more of these:

1. Exercises for range of motion These are designed to increase one's flexibility. The Arthritis Foundation recommends a some range of motion exercises to the hip, shoulder knees, hips, and ankles. In order not to violate any copyright laws, we encourage readers to visit the web site of the US Arthritis Foundation at http://www.arthritis.org/conditions/exercise/def ault.asp. Go to the section "conditions as well as treatments" above the homepage. The right and left hand columns have exercises for OA patients can perform.

2. Strengthening exercises - these workouts are designed to strengthen muscles around joints. They can aid in improving joint motion. Exercises for strengthening can be isometric or isotonic. Isometric exercises strengthen (contract) the muscles with no joint movements. Isotonic exercises are performed against resistance , such as an unweighted object or against any resistance from your body weight. Also, the Arthritis

Foundation has examples of these exercises , which they go over in depth.

3. Aerobic exercises help improve lung and heart function and aid to maintain the proper body weight. Also known as endurance exercises These exercises must be performed for at least thirty minutes three times per week.

Patients who suffer from OA might not be able jog or play tennis, or participate in sports like football, but they could find a sport they'd enjoy. Through trial and error, arthritis patients can choose the appropriate sport for them. The best practice is to choose exercises that don't strain the joints that are affected by OA and have little impact. Doctor. Donald Grelsamer names the following activities that are suitable for OA patients: if the upper extremities like shoulders and elbows suffer, patients may take part in running, swimming ski, cross-country skiing, walking, hiking, bicycling as well as aquatic exercise. [17]

If the cervical and back vertebrae are affected, they are able to take a swim or do aquatic exercises. In the event that you have lower extremities (hips or ankles, knees, and knees) have been affected patients are able to exercise in the water, swim row golf, cycle on stationary bikes and canoe. [18]

The negative side effects of over-training

Humans are prone to do over-the-top things. If people who suffer from OA cannot endure discomfort, they do everything they can to bring more value of their lives. It doesn't matter if it's strenuous exercises or stretching OA sufferers are prone to forgetting and overdo their workouts in the fear that not working out enough can cause greater discomfort.

What are the signs of training too much? It is suggested that the Canadian Arthritis Society mentions some symptoms of overtraining.19

Feelings of indifference, sadness, restlessness, or irritability

• Decreased self-confidence

* Anxiety and emotional instability

* Sleep problems

* A decreased appetite or weight loss

* Risk of injury

* Soreness and pain the muscle

* Unable to meet the training goals

Natural Treatment vs Medical Treatment for OA

There's little distinction between medical and the natural treatment options for RA as well as OA. Doctors generally have almost identical views when discussing the natural and medical treatment in RA as well as OA.

Dr. Grelsamer states that the drugs that are used for treating OA are of three varieties: [20Dr. Grelsamer says that the drugs used to treat OA consist of three

*Aspirin (and its closest relatives)

* Acetaminophen (Tylenol, etc)

* NSAIDs

The decision to prescribe a drug will depend on the doctor's view of the patient's OA and other health issues, and the patient's response to the drug. It is normal to expect that some patients can successfully adapt to the medication that is prescribed, while others do not. Due to their chemical composition they can cause severe adverse effects for certain. OA patients should report these adverse effects to their physicians so that they can suggest a solution or changed in the dosage or reducing the dosage and frequency.

The surgical intervention, which is a component of the treatment plan for OA has prompted a great deal of research in health institutions. For instance, the Cleveland Clinic, for instance is home to more than 30 principal investigators who collaborate alongside scientists from the Cleveland Clinic Lerner Research Institute.

There are more than 100 clinical and research trials taking place in The Cleveland Clinic so that an understanding of the treatment of musculoskeletal conditions is achievable. Researchers are working towards improvements in joint replacement procedures and other orthopaedic procedures that can improve your quality of life OA patients. [21]

The research projects that are related to joint replacement are:

* Regeneration and healing of cartilage by using tissue engineering repair techniques

* Utilization Adult stem cells to aid in cartilage repair

* Study of the degeneration of cartilage in arthritis and other conditions,

Amount of cement that is used for hip replacement and the way it affects the artificial joint's life and function.

Evaluation of the impact of the artificial joint design and how the body refuses or accepts implants

* Identifying the most effective medication to prevent blood clots following joint surgery.

* Assessment of new techniques for knee and hip joint surgery.

* Improvement in surgical techniques that connect muscle and bone to artificial knee and hip joints.

In terms of natural remedies are concerned, the same natural ingredients like glucosamine and omega-3 fatty acids vinegar and honey (vinegar and honey) for natural treatment isn't new and is considered an old-fashioned remedy.

In actual fact, Hippocrates used them to treat various ailments more than two thousand years ago.) are listed. It is recommended to supplement (Vitamins C and B complex, E, boron, copper Boswellia Devil's claw zinc, selenium, and iron are recommended; as is manganese and diverse homeopathic herbs and plants are also suggested in OA patients. [23]

In addition to going the extra mile to deal with OA Dr. Ronald Lawrence also encourages OA sufferers to explore the acupuncture method (ideally the frequency should be once per month, but at least two or three times per year could be beneficial) and chriropractic therapies (to correct structural imbalances that can affect the functioning in the spinal column) Massage (OA patients have been reported to feel better after a massage) and a method known as Rolfing.

Rolfing was first introduced through the Dr. Ida Rolf who is biochemist at the Rockefeller Institute. It's a proven method of bodywork (typically 10-15 sessions) that is designed to relieve tension and chronic stress. [24]

Chapter 6: Gout

What exactly is Gout?

As per the Cleveland Clinic, gout is a type of arthritis that is characterised by acute and sudden pain, redness, tenderness and swelling (inflammation) in certain joints. It typically affects just only one joint at a.

The region most often affected is the toe that is larger however gout may affect other joints of the leg, such as knees or ankle, foot. It is less common in the arms , wrist, hand and elbow. The fingers are not often affected, while the spine is rarely affected. [1]

What are the signs of Gout?

* Instant severe joint pain that usually occurs in the first hour of the day

* Joint that's swollen and soft to touch.

* Skin that is red or purple around the joint[22

What causes Gout?

Many believed that only the wealthy and famous suffer from Gout, due to their well-known drinking and food habits. Although drinking and eating too much could cause the formation of gout, they're not the main cause of the symptoms. [3]

Gout occurs because there are abnormal accumulations in sodium urate crystals inside the joint cartilage. These are then released into the joint fluid. Uric acid crystals can also be responsible for the development of kidney stones.

It is formed by the uric acid that is a natural chemical found in the human body. Uric acid, in turn, is produced by the natural degrading of DNA and RNA (the DNA in cells). Uric acid is found in large quantities in certain food items, including seafood, red meats and anchovies.

In normal quantities the uric acid is dissolving in blood and it easily moves through the kidneys, and eventually becomes waste. In excess, however, it can could make people more susceptible to developing gout. [4]

It is not the case that all people who has excessive levels of uric acids will develop Gout. The capacity of kidneys to remove uric acid is a large part influenced by genetics. The most important thing to keep in the mind is that if one person in the family has Gout, it doesn't necessarily mean that the other members of the family is likely to develop the illness.

Gout attacks are frequent and occur within the same joint. They can last for a few days or two weeks, unless treated. [5]

In the course of it is possible that attacks become more frequent, involving joints other than the one and causing more severe symptoms with a longer time. The result could cause injury in the joint.

Although some patients will suffer one attack, about 90% of those suffering from one Gout attack will experience at least one more, however, it might not happen for many years following the first attack. Other patients may experience attacks on a regular basis. [6]

Over one million Americans suffer from Gout, especially among males older than 40, obese drinking alcohol, and those who take tablets to control blood pressure. Gout can also affect women, however they are generally women who have reached menopausal stage.

Medical Treatment for Gout

It is impossible to cure gout however, it is treatable and managed. The symptoms typically disappear within 24 hours of the treatment is started. [7]

Gout treatment is a medical procedure to ease inflammation and pain and reduce the risk of any future attacks that may result in joint injuries. The type of treatment is contingent on the age of the patient as well as the medications the patient is taking, his medical history , and the severity of an individual's attacks. Medicines are commonly used to treat Gout. They include:

Anti-inflammatory medications - the medicines are taken until the attack is over. If adverse effects develop it is possible to alter the medications.

Nonsteroidal anti-inflammatory medications (NSAIDs) These are prescribed to treat painful and sudden attacks.

Corticosteroids (also known as steroids) can also used for those who do not have the ability to use

NSAIDs. Steroids can reduce inflammation and are instilled into joints or taken as pills.

Colchicine - often prescribed long-term in low doses in order to lower the chance of having repeated attacks. [8]

According to the Cleveland Clinic says that dietary changes for the majority of people do not contribute significantly to managing high levels of uric acid within the body. However restricting certain foods that trigger an increase in the production of uric acid as well as cutting down on alcohol consumption could help relieve symptoms and lessen the intensity and frequency of attacks.

The Natural Way to Treat Gout

The primary goal of the natural method is on diet and food.

Food & Diet

People suffering from gout are advised to put in an effort to achieve the below objectives:

1. Eliminate alcohol. Alcohol increases acid production and decreases the body's ability to

eliminate urine, which may cause kidney dysfunction. The doctor Dr. Murray quotes Petersford et and Harrison in Harrison's Principles of Internal Medicine that for many people, removing alcohol by itself is enough to decrease the amount of uric acids and thus reduce the risk of developing Gout. [9]

(2) Follow the diet with a low purine content and high levels of purine should be avoided. This is achieved by avoiding organ meat and shellfish, meat as well as yeast (brewer's and baker's), mackerel, herring and sardines and anchovies. [10]

(3) Maintain an ideal weight. People with gout attacks typically are overweight and have higher risk of developing heart disease. Losing a significant amount of pounds may decrease the amount of serum uric acids.

(4) Eat complex carbs, decrease calories and decrease intake of protein Dr. Murray recommends gout patients to avoid refined carbs and saturated fats since carbohydrates can increase the production of uric acid and fats

hinder the elimination of the uric acid. Protein consumption should be moderate.

(5) Drink plenty of fluids as they dilute urine, which lowers the risk of developing kidney stones. They also help in the elimination process.

(6) Increase intake of flavonoids. Studies have found that eating an equivalent of half a pound of fresh cherries daily aids in lowering the levels of uric acid. The richest sources of flavonoid compounds are hawthorne berries, cherries blueberries, dark-red/blue fruit. They also seem to reduce damage to joints, and their significance can be seen in their capacity to stop the degradation of collagen.

Supplements Nutritional for the Treatment of Gout

Making changes to our diets should be enough for treating gout. Doctor. Murray says that adding nutritional supplements isn't required. The most common suggestion is to use a multi vitamin or a multi mineral formulas that meet RDA requirements.

If patients decide to go to supplementation due to a variety of reasons the doctor. Murray advises quercetin, omega-3 oils, and Folic acid.

Quercetin has a role that is like the drug called allopurinol. It reduces the production of uric acids and also the release of inflammatory chemicals. Vegetables and fruits are fantastic suppliers of quercetin. For the best results, a dosage of 200-400 milligrams of quercetin should be taken along with bromelain between meals, three times a day.

Omega-3 oils inhibit the production of substances known as leukotrienes which are the primary triggers for tissue injury and inflammation.

Folic acid blocks the production of xanthine the enzyme responsible for generating the uric acid. While it is not proven scientifically as a reliable treatment for gout, there are positive outcomes that show the benefits it can provide to patients suffering from Gout. A dosage of 10-40 milligrams a day is suggested.

Patients who want to take Folic acid should discuss the matter with their doctor because the high levels of folic acid have been reported to interfere with some medications and cover up the symptoms of a Vitamin B-12 deficiency.

Plant-based medicines in the treatment of Gout

Exercises to Treat Gout

When the patient's gout problem is controlled, exercises to strengthen the joint affected and maintain an appropriate weight must be done.

Similar to rheumatoid arthritis and osteoarthritis, three kinds of exercises are required:

* Exercises in range of motion to increase joint flexibility (example moving the foot, starting from the ankle's point by making circular movements),

Strengthening exercises that make muscle stronger (example resistance exercises such as lifting small weights),

* Exercises for endurance to keep the heart stronger and keep your body weight at a healthy level. Examples include swimming, walking and cycling.

The standard approach to every exercise plan is to speak with your physical therapist and physician first.

Patients may also take steps to safeguard their joints. Exercises should be done in a safe manner in order to avoid putting pressure on joints. A proper rest period between workouts is a good idea. Making use of equipment such as carts, grab bars or canes will reduce the pressure on your joints.

It is the Canadian Arthritis Society says that there are three options to safeguard joints that include Pacing (alternating difficult or repeated chores with simpler ones) and repositioning the joint in a way it can be utilized without creating unnecessary streets, avoid settling in one place for long periods of time and the use of aids that make the daily work simpler. [11]

Relaxation, breathing correctly yoga, meditation, and visualization can help patients feel they're in better control over their conditions. As time passes, they are able how to manage their condition and can return to their normal routine.

Chapter 7: Living With Rheumatoid Arthritis

If you've been diagnosed with RA If you are diagnosed with RA, it is important to be aware of how you can control general health. Being aware of your overall health could enhance your RA symptoms too. Therapy for RA is designed to decrease inflammation of joints as well as relieve pain. It also helps to reduce the disability that it causes as well as reduce joint damage and deformity, and slow in the progression of damage or deformity to joints. With the assistance of occupational therapists and physical therapists, patients can learn to safeguard their joints. Surgery may be necessary based on the extent of joint injury.

Drugs

In the beginning phases of the disease doctors will prescribe medicines which have the least amount of adverse negative effects. As the disease advances, stronger drugs may be required. Each medication is liable to cause side negative effects. The list of all side consequences of RA drugs is difficult because various drugs can cause different reactions to different medications.

* Nonsteroidal anti-inflammatory medications (NAIDs) These are prescribed for pain relief as well as to decrease the inflammation (e.g., Advil or Motrin). These drugs do not slow down the progress to the diagnosis. If taken in large doses over a long time they could cause complications. The side effects could include:

or Edema (swelling of feet)

A higher chance of suffering from bruises

o Hypertension

A Kidney injury

o Liver damage

O Heartburn

Stomach upsets and stomach ulcers

O Tinnitus - ringing within the ears

Potentially increased chances of developing blood clots and heart attacks or stroke

* Corticosteroids can be used to lessen the pain and inflammation as well as in slowing joint injuries. They are generally prescribed after the NSAIDs are not helping. If the patient is suffering from only one joint inflamed and the doctor decides to inject the steroids directly in the joint. Corticosteroids provide quick relief which lasts for weeks to months, based on the degree and severity of symptoms. Common side effects include:

O Cataracts

o Glaucoma

Obtained blood fats that are elevated and levels of blood sugar

O Face with a round shape

o Weight gain

o An increase in appetite

o Bone loss

Muscle weakness

The skin is thinned.

* Antirheumatic medications that are disease-modifying (DMARDs) This drug could slow down the progress of the disease and protect against permanent damage to joints as well as other tissues. The earlier the patient starts taking a medication the more effective it is. It can take anywhere from six to four months before a patient can begin to feel the effects. It is crucial to continue using it even when it does not seem to work initially. There are some side effects that can occur.

o Stomach upset

o Greater susceptibility to infection

o Bone Marrow

o Lung infections (severe)

* Immunosuppressant. As RA is an auto-immune illness suppression of the immune system can help reduce the destruction to healthy tissues. These drugs are prescribed to ease stiffness in the morning, pain and tender or swollen joints. It is common to see results within 2 weeks of beginning the treatment. The most common side effects include:

Infusion site reactions, such as redness and swelling

Risk of developing serious infections

A blood disorder

o Congestive heart failure

If the medicine you take makes you feel nauseated or causes you to have nausea, consider having it in conjunction with food. The NSAIDs you take daily are best taken in the evening or afternoon rather than in the morning. If they still cause stomach discomfort, you can take it with a medicine which reduces stomach acid. When you're on a DMA and it causes stomach pain consult your physician to determine for a change to an injection version.

Certain NSAIDs cause stomach ulcers. Avoid drinking alcohol as alcohol in combination with NSAIDs may increase the amount of gastric bleeding. It is also recommended to stay clear of other medicines that contain NSAID such as some over-the-counter cold remedies.

Corticosteroid is a cause of insomnia. To fight this, you should you should take a dose once a day in the morning. Avoid stimulants such as caffeine, which can cause insomnia.

The use of antidepressants as well as narcotic analgesics create dry and irritated mouths. Soak the mouth using sugar-free chewing gum or hard candy. You can also try sucking on ice chips. Beware of alcohol-based mouthwashes and alcohol-containing mouthwashes which can cause dry mouth to get worse.

If your medication causes mouth ulcers, try to avoid spicy or salty foods. The excessive consumption of citrus fruits could cause irritation to mouth ulcers.

Occupational Therapy

A therapist who is occupational can teach the patient how to perform routine tasks that don't strain joints that are painful. For instance, if it is difficult to open a door because of pain in the arms, leaning onto the door might be a good alternative to pushing the door using arms.

Surgery

The doctor might recommend surgery if the treatments mentioned haven't been successful. The procedure aims to fix the joint and make it functional again. The surgical procedure can assist in correcting deformities as well as decrease the pain. These are some of the options for surgical procedures:

* Arthroplasty is a total reconstruction of the joint. The damaged joints are removed, and a new joint (prosthesis) composed of steel and plastic is placed.

Tendon repair surgery could help repair loose or ruptured tendons in the joint.

* Synovectomy. This is the elimination of the joint liner if the liner around the joint (synovium) is painful and inflamed.

* If the option of arthroplasty isn't available then the joint can be surgically fixed to encourage an osteo-fibrillation.

Staying Active

You are able to and should exercise if you suffer from RA. It is essential to exercise to alleviate pain and boost your energy levels. It also lowers the chance of developing diseases such as diabetes and heart disease. Before beginning an exercise routine talk to your doctor or physical therapist to determine the right workout routine for you. The ideal program would consist of aerobic exercise to increase the strength of your lungs and heart. Additionally, you will be doing exercises that strengthen your muscles stronger, so that they can support your joints better. Exercises for stretching are essential to ensure that your muscles remain flexible and joints in motion. If you're not yet accustomed to exercising begin slowly until you are able to build up your fitness and endurance. Don't overdo it. In the end, you will be able to work out longer and harder. Pay attention to your body's signals while working out. If a joint gets painful, take it off and then work on different muscles. Reduce your exercise routine when you notice the increase of joint discomfort.

People suffering from RA might be at higher risk of losing muscle. Nearly half of RA sufferers experience loss of muscle mass as well as an increased fat weight. This can cause an infection, fatigue and even the possibility of disability. This risk can be reduced by performing resistance training. You can perform resistance exercises using small dumbbells as well as rubber exercise tubing and water bottles.

Here are the advantages that you can gain by doing resistance training

Training for resistance with high intensity could decrease arthritis pain by 53% according to an article that was published in Journal of Clinical Rheumatology.

* Resistance exercise, performed at least two times per week, will help improve your flexibility and help you get used to doing everyday tasks such as walking, climbing steps , and getting up from your chair.

* In conjunction with cardiovascular exercise resistance training may increase blood flow and provide an increase in cardiovascular health. This is essential for RA patients with higher risks of developing heart disease.

Fatigue and Pain

Here are simple solutions to alleviate pain without medication. They can be used on their own or in conjunction with one the other.

* Cold and hot treatments The use of heat can be beneficial to treat chronic pain. Cold packs offer relief from acute pain. Apply the pack directly on the site of pain. If hot treatments offer relief better than those that are cold, then you can try any of the following methods.

You can take a long and very warm shower the first thing at the beginning of your day. The steam from the shower helps to reduce stiffness.

To soak in an icy bath. The pain will ease when you are immersed in warm.

o Purchase a moist heating pad at the drugstore, or make it yourself by warming a moist washcloth in the microwave oven for 1 minute. Wrap the hot pad in a towel before placing it on the area affected in the 15-20 minutes.

To ease joint pain on the hands apply mineral oil, then wear rubber gloves. Your hands should be submerged in the tap for 5-10 minutes.

* Exercise regularly - Keep your joints and muscles active can ease the pain. It can also increase your overall fitness level.

Relaxation techniques such as deep breaths, guided imagery, visualization as well as other relaxation techniques will help you train your muscles to let go.

* Massages - Massages are a great way to ease muscles and relax tension.

* Topical lotions - Topical creams that are applied directly on the joints and muscles that are painful may reduce the sensitiveness to pain.

* Acupuncture is the method of inserting needles in the body along specific points to ease pain.

Positive attitude and an enlightened sense of humor can help distract your brain from experiencing discomfort. Do your best to not be angry even when you are feeling discomfort. Instead, focus on positive thoughts.

Alongside fatigue, pain is the most commonly reported and problematic sign of RA. The constant battle with pain, all day long it can make you tired and lead to fatigue. Being tired however could aggravate discomfort and cause it to become harder to manage. The reason for fatigue is the condition itself. The inflammatory cytokines, blood proteins which are released when you suffer from arthritis are similar to those that are released when you get the flu. The presence of inflammation typically results in fatigue. If there's no inflammation or the treatment for inflammation isn't bringing down fatigue, it could be due to one of the following possible causes:

* Side effects of medication Some medicines are associated with fatigue. This includes antidepressants and blood pressure medications insomnia aids and painkillers and even some non-steroidal anti-inflammatory medications. Corticosteriods are a great way to keep you awake during the late at night and can cause fatigue.

* Fatigue resulting from anemia that occurs in RA is often caused by anemia. The anemia could be the result of an ulcer in the intestines caused through medications or by an underlying disease.

* Sleeplessness - If the pain is keeping you awake in the night, it can result in daytime fatigue.

* Depression - The illness can take away your ability to fully enjoy your everyday activities and result in depression. If you're suffering from depression there are hormonal changes.

* Other medical conditions Your fatigue could be due to other medical conditions you are suffering from.

The treatment for fatigue is to treat the root cause. Based on the root nature of the issue, your doctor can recommend the appropriate treatment. There are , however, things you can accomplish yourself.

* Move around An exercise program that is guided can greatly help RA patients. Endorphins release can increase energy levels and help improve the quality of sleep at night.

* Pacing - Divide activities throughout the day, allowing the body to rest between work.

Ask for help if you're struggling to complete certain chores, try asking for assistance.

Making it Through The Day with RA

Being able to get through the day when you suffer from RA frequently demands energy that you do not have, and can cause discomfort that you are unable to live with. Here are some ways to keep your life on track despite the discomfort and fatigue:

Begin your day with a the luxury of a warm, long shower. Joints can feel stiff and stiff after an extended period of inactivity. A warm and long shower can help. Stretching can help loosen tight joints.

* Many RA patients feel more energetic early in the day. If this is the case for you, plan important tasks earlier in the morning so that you're able to finish them.

In the event that your position requires you to sit standing for long durations, think about purchasing a floor mat with padding or sit on stool, if you can. If you work from a desk all day, make sure to stand every now and again in order to move your muscles.

* If you are sitting for long periods be sure that the setup is ergonomically appropriate. Be sure that your posture improves performance and reduces the pain. The computer's monitor is best placed at eye level. Your feet must be flat in the flooring. Your chair should be able to help your back.

* If you're feeling exhausted, you can take cat napping. They'll give you energy to make it throughout the entire day.

Don't speed through your work. Give yourself at least a half hour allowance for the necessary errands. So, you don't feel exhausted, stressed or overwhelmed.

* Be smart in doing your errands. In the supermarket, you can get the service of a delivery to bring your bags back to your car. Get help taking your items off. If you aren't enough to go to the shop, go on the internet instead.

The intensity of your symptoms may vary from day to day. Tell your loved ones the severity of your condition by using a numeric scale ranging from zero (no feeling) and up (worst discomfort). You can tell them, "Today, I'm at 9 and cannot take my children to school. Do you have the time to help me?"

* Sleep well. Develop a bedtime routine that you can get your body into sleeping in a regular time.

Chapter 8: Reversing Rheumatoid Arthritis

They claim it is because RA is a chronic disease that is incurable and it will only get worse as you the passage of time. If you are confirmed to have the condition you'll be on medications to treat the symptoms. However, there are indications that medication isn't the only option to treat RA. Natural methods, when combined with conventional treatments, can aid patients to manage their illness.

The best way to treat RA does not focus on the symptoms, but rather the root cause of the illness. The most common cause of RA is an infection with a bacterium that is concealed inside the cell. The infection is triggered in the event that your immune system weak condition. Another reason for RA is the increase in nutritional deficiencies. RA is an illness of the immune system. When the immune system gets stronger by diet and nutrition, symptoms of RA will be reduced dramatically.

Rheumatoid Arthritis Diet

The most effective approach to eating for people suffering from RA is to follow a well-balanced and balanced diet that is focused on foods that are plant-based. Around two-thirds of a diet should be based on vegetables, fruits as well as whole grain. The rest should be low-fat or fat-free dairy products as well as lean sources of protein. Although there isn't a specific "diet" which RA patients must adhere to Researchers have identified certain food items that could aid in reducing inflammation. They are a large portion of the "Mediterranean Diet" which focuses on vegetables, fish and olive oil.

Foods that fight RA include:

* Certain types of fish such as herring, mackerel, trout, salmon, tuna, sardines, anchovies and other cold-water fish are rich in inflammation-fighting omega-3 fatty acids which reduce inflammatory proteins in the body. They are able to ease joint pain and ease stiffness during the

morning. It is recommended to consume at least 3-4 ounces every two days.

* The fruits and vegetables are rich in antioxidants, which help boost the immune system and aid in fighting inflammation. The most recommended ones are blueberries, cherries, blackberries, strawberries as well as spinach, kale, and broccoli. It is recommended to consume at least 1.5 to 2 cups fruits as well as 2 to 3 cups veggies each meal.

* Nuts are full of inflammation-fighting monounsaturated fat, protein and fiber. They are a must-have snack when you're looking to shed some weight. Consume 1.5 teaspoons of nuts per day and select from walnuts and pine nuts, as well as pistachios and almonds.

* Beans contain a variety of antioxidants and anti-inflammatory substances. They also are a great source of protein, fiber as well as folic acid as well as minerals like iron, magnesium zinc, potassium and magnesium. The most effective choices are pinto red kidney, black and Garbanzo beans. You should eat a cup twice per week.

* Olive oil is rich in antioxidants and monounsaturated fats that are heart-healthy. Additionally, it has oleocanthal which is a chemical that reduces the pain and inflammation. The extra-virgin olive oil can be considered the most effective option because it's less refined and refined. It has more nutrients in it than other types made from olive oil. It is recommended to use 2 to 3 tablespoons daily for cooking and salad dressing.

* Onions are rich in antioxidants beneficial to the body. They also can lower inflammation, increase the risk of cardiovascular disease as well as bad cholesterol. Include them in salads or sandwiches, sauteed dishes, as well as in stir-fries.

* Fiber decreases C-reactive proteins (CRP) CRP is a substance found in blood that signals inflammation. Consuming fiber in foods is more effective than supplementing with fiber for the reduction of CRP levels. Carotenoids-rich foods are particularly good for lowering CRP. One of these is peppers and carrots.

Certain research suggests that the chemicals found in cherries can aid in reducing pain and inflammation. A study indicates it that RA sufferers who consumed 8oz of cherries daily over a period of several weeks experienced positive improvements on their levels of pain. They also saw an improvement in the inflammation and stiffness.

* Eastern medical practices have relied on ginger to ease inflammation and pain in the joints. Fresh ginger is the best option and contains the most chemicals that have medicinal properties that boost the immune system.

* Pineapples contain bromelain an enzyme that helps reduce inflammation as well as ease stiffness and pain that is that are associated with RA. Freshly squeezed and fresh juice from pineapples are the most effective sources of this enzyme.

* Turmeric is a spice which has been used for a long time to aid in the relief of pain and inflammation. It's much more effective when it is used in conjunction with bromelain. Turmeric can be used to cook with.

RA patients must avoid these foods which can cause inflammation:

* Hamburger and various other types of meat that has been grilled or baked at a high temperatures. Advanced glycation end products (AGE) is a toxin which is produced when food items are cooked and grilled, or fried, or pasteurized. The AGEs destroy certain proteins in the body, and the body breaks them down through cytokines, which are messengers of inflammation. Reduce the amount of AGE by avoiding food cooked in extremely high temperatures.

The Omega-6 Fatty Acids are found in sunflower, corn cottonseed, soybean, and safflower oils. They can cause inflammation. Replace them with omega-3 options like olive oil, flax seeds, nuts, as well as pumpkin seeds.

It has been associated to inflammation and intestinal irritation. Even though its role in RA is sparse, studies show that gluten-free diets increase levels of inflammation-fighting antibodies.

* Refined sugar triggers the blood sugar to increase. The high blood sugar levels can trigger the production of inflammatory substances that

could cause joint pain. Avoid sweets, processed food white flour baked goods and sodas.

* Foods processed are rich in unhealthy fats that can cause inflammation. Stay away from chips, cookies as well as other processed snacks. Instead, choose fresh fruits.

* Dairy products can cause pain in arthritis because of the kind of protein they have. They can cause irritation to the tissue around joints. Instead of getting protein from dairy, take the nutrients from vegetables.

The majority of canned foods are packed with sodium, which may cause blood pressure to rise. If you have to eat canned foods, make sure you choose lower sodium options.

* Salt can cause fluid retention, which is just one of many reasons which can cause high blood pressure. Be aware that corticosteroids, a RA drug causes the body to hold more sodium. Be careful when you use salt or try to stay clear of it in any way you can.

Nutrient-rich food items that could be Medicine

Three essential nutrients are vital for arthritis treatment. These nutrients perform functions ranging from slowing the loss of cartilage and reducing the out of control immune system.

* Omega-3 PUFAs - Excellent source of the nutrient include coldwater fish, as well as specific seeds and nuts, like walnuts and soybean kernels. Studies conducted by scientists demonstrate this nutrient's capacity to dramatically reduce joint tenderness. It decreases the duration of stiffness in the morning, reduces discomfort and enhances functional capability. Omega-3 PUFAs protect against atherosclerosis which is the hardening of arteries.

* Selenium A good source of Selenium are whole-grain wheat and shellfish such as crabs and oysters. Selenium is a trace mineral with antioxidant properties. It can be beneficial in preventing arthritis and other diseases such as age-related blindness heart disease, cancer kidney disease, and cataracts.

* Vitamin D Recent studies suggest that, in addition to protecting against osteoporosis and other diseases, vitamin D might be useful for RA

also. It could be an immunosuppressant that is a treatment for RA. Fortified foods like eggs, breads fortified with vitamin D and cereals , and milk are excellent sources of vitamin D.

Arthritis Food Myths

If you search on the internet, you'll find some foods that are claimed to be able of reducing or even causing RA symptoms. These include:

Myth: A dozen gin-soaked raises a day could provide relief from pain that is natural.

To keep their color it is treated with sulfur dioxide as they are processed. In the past 25 years researchers discovered that a sulfur-containing substance called dimethyl sulfoxide could help lessen damaging joint changes that mice experience. The findings were not conclusive at the very least, but these studies support the idea that raisins' sulfur content has anti-inflammatory properties. In the end, there is no evidence-based basis to this myth.

Myth: Drinking vinegar from the cider can ease discomfort.

There is a claim that beta-carotene contained in apple cider vinegar eliminates free radicals that are present in the body which ravage our immune system. It is also claimed that the vinegar breaks down the acid crystals that cause stiff joints, and removes them and out of your body. Gout is the only type of arthritis that has acid crystals. Cider vinegar does not relieve pain caused by gout.

Myths - Dairy products cause arthritis to get worse.

There was a study that put RA patients on a dairy-free diet or on placebo diets. Those on the special diet were no better that those on the placebo. The bottom line is, for very few people, limiting dairy products may help bring down RA symptoms but it could be because, to a degree, they are lactose-intolerant. Dairy products are therefore safe to most RA patients.

• Myth – Nightshade vegetables aggravate arthritis.

Tomatoes, potatoes, eggplants and peppers are among those that fall in the nightshade category. They all contain a chemical called solanine which has been pointed as a culprit in arthritis pain. This claim is not backed by any research. In fact, there are researches that suggest these vegetables may actually help reduce the symptoms. People with RA may actually benefit from these vegetables.

• Myth – A low-acid diet lessens arthritis pain.

No formal research has been done on this. Any food, when it reaches the stomach, is bathed in hydrochloric acid. Whatever food you eat, whether low acid or not, will not affect the blood's optimal pH of 7.4. Other compounds act on the food particles you consumed to reach the proper pH before the nutrients are absorbed in the bloodstream. This happens automatically no matter what your food choices are.

• Myth – A raw food diet relieves symptoms.

There are positive effects on a raw food diet. In a 1990's study, those on a raw food diet reported more relief from RA symptoms compared to those on a traditional diet. The positive effects weren't measurable though when it comes to disease activity in RA. There were no measurable benefits on morning stiffness, pain at rest and pain on movement. The raw food eaters even experienced nausea and diarrhea during the diet. The bottom line is eating uncooked fruits and vegetables are good as long as you do it in moderation to avoid stomach discomfort. When it comes to RA, raw food diet delivers no particular relief.

• Myth – You can drink as much red wine as you want.

Moderate amounts of red wine may bring about good health benefits from protecting the heart to reducing illnesses. Excessive wine consumption is not recommended. It may even react negatively with your arthritis medication.

• Myth – Gelatin strengthens joints.

Gelatin contains collagen, one of the materials that make up joint cartilage. It seems logical therefore that consuming gelatin will strengthen your joints because you add collagen to them. There is no scientific study that can back this up, however. Besides, gelatin doesn't travel intact to a particular part of the body. When digested, its components are used for tissues, enzymes and various biological processes.

- Myth – Citrus fruits causes inflammation.

There are claims that citrus fruits promote inflammation. This is not true. On the contrary, vitamin C is critical in the formation of collagen and proteoglycans – the major components of cartilage. Vitamin C is also an antioxidant that can quench free radicals.

- Myth – Fasting relieves RA pain.

A research found that fasting can improve RA symptoms; however, too much fasting can undermine the immune system. When it comes to food, the better way to get relief from RA symptoms is to lose excess weight with a healthy diet.

Dietary Changes to ease Rheumatoid Arthritis Pain

- Shed extra pounds – Create an eating plan that will help you shed off excess weight. Doing so will take the pressure off your joints. It will also improve the quality of life. A study shows that normal weight people with RA, even those who are just slightly overweight, have a better quality of life compared to those who are obese.

•   Consider going vegetarian – One study found that RA patients who turned vegetarian or vegan reported an improvement in their RA symptoms, including pain score, morning stiffness and grip strength. Vegetarian or vegan diets can be restrictive though so some have difficulty staying in it. If you cannot give up meat, the best thing to do is to add more greens in your plate. The antioxidants you will get from them will do you wonders.

•   Find out about allergies - Food allergies, particularly to dairy and shrimp, may aggravate RA. You may try elimination diets which involves removing all potential allergens then slowly reintroducing them to see which one trigger symptoms.

Chapter 9: Rheumatoid Arthritis-Friendly Recipes

Lemon Rosemary Chicken

Ingredients:

4 6-oz boneless, skinless chicken breasts, halved

2 t extra-virgin olive oil

1 t salt-free lemon-pepper seasoning

1 t salt-free citrus-herb seasoning

Salt (optional)

3 organic lemons, thinly sliced

Fresh rosemary sprigs

1 ¼ cup organic chicken broth

½ t crushed garlic

Directions:

1.   Preheat oven to 375 degrees F.

2.   Brush both sides of chicken pieces with olive oil and sprinkle with lemon-pepper seasoning, citrus-herb seasoning and salt (optional). Set aside.

3.   In a baking dish, arrange 2 to 3 slices of lemon and a sprig of rosemary for each chicken piece.

4.   Place chicken, smooth sides up, on lemon and rosemary. Top each with another sprig of rosemary and 2 to 3 slices of lemon.

5.   Bake in the oven for 20 to 25 minutes or until chicken is no longer pink.

6.   Remove chicken to platter and cover with aluminum foil to keep warm.

7.   In a small saucepan, combine half of the rosemary from the baking dish and any brown bits.

8.   Add chicken broth and garlic.

9.   Bring to a boil over medium-heat. Cook until mixture is reduced by half.

10.   Using a fine-mesh strainer, strain the mixture to discard the solids.

11.   Serve the mixture with chicken. Garnish with additional lemon slices and rosemary sprigs.

Mediterranean Vegetables

Ingredients:

1 package (16 oz) loose-pack frozen mixed vegetables (broccoli, cauliflower, carrots)

1 can (14.5 oz) diced tomatoes with basil, garlic and oregano

1 T capers, drained

Directions:

1.   In a microwave-safe bowl, combine frozen mixed vegetables, tomatoes and drained capers. Cover with plastic wrap.

2.   Microwave on high setting for 6 to 8 minutes, stirring halfway through the cooking time.

Note: Be creative when it comes to mixing vegetables. Great mixtures include baby peas, baby carrots, snow peas and baby corn or Brussels sprouts, cauliflower and carrots.

Cherry Quinoa Porridge

Ingredients:

1 cup water

½ cup dry quinoa

½ cup dried unsweetened cherries

½ t vanilla extract

¼ t ground cinnamon

1 T honey, optional

Directions:

1.   In a medium-sized saucepan, stir together the first five ingredients and bring to a boil over medium-high heat.

2.   Reduce heat and simmer covered for 15 minutes or until all the water has been absorbed and the quinoa is tender.

3.   Drizzle with honey before serving.

Pumpkin Soup

Ingredients:

1 cup chopped onion

1 1-inch piece ginger, peeled and minced

1 clove garlic, minced

6 cups vegetable stock, divided

4 cups pumpkin puree

1 t salt

½ t chopped fresh thyme

½ cup half-and-half

1 t chopped fresh parsley

Directions:

1.   In a large soup pot, cook onions, garlic and ginger in ½ cup vegetable stock. Let it simmer for about 5 minutes.

2.   Add pumpkin puree, the remaining 5 ½ vegetable stock, salt and thyme. Cook for 30 minutes.

3.   Using a handheld blender, puree soup until smooth.

4.   Remove soup from heat and stir in half-and-half.

5.   Sprinkle chopped parsley before serving.

Poached Eggs with Curried Vegetables

Ingredients:

2 t extra -virgin olive oil

1 large onion, chopped

2 cloves garlic, minced

1 T yellow curry powder

½ lb sliced button mushrooms

2 med zucchinis, diced

1 14-oz can chickpeas, drained

1 cup water

1/8 t crushed red pepper (optional)

½ t white vinegar

4 large eggs

Directions:

1.   In a large nonstick skilled, sauté onions for 5 minutes or until translucent.

2.   Add garlic and cook for 30 seconds.

3.   Stir in curry powder and cook for 2 minutes.

4.   Add mushrooms and cook until they have released their liquid and are tender.

5.   Add zucchini, chickpeas, water and red pepper (if using) and bring to a boil.

6.   Reduce heat and simmer covered for 15 to 20 minutes or until zucchini is tender.

7.   Meanwhile, add water to a depth of 3 inches in a large saucepan. Bring to a boil. Reduce heat. Add vinegar and maintain a light simmer.

8.   Crack eggs and gently slip into the water, one at a time, and as close as possible to the surface of the water. Simmer for 3 to 5 minutes. Remove eggs with a slotted spoon.

Kippers Salad

Ingredients:

½ cup reduced-fat mayonnaise

1 small onion, finely chopped

1 celery stalk, finely chopped

1 T chopped fresh parsley

1 t lemon juice

1 clove garlic, minced

1/8 t salt

1/8 t ground black pepper

1 6-oz can kippers, drained

Directions:

1.   In a medium-sized bowl, stir together the first eight ingredients.

2.   Add flaked kippers and gently toss to combine.

3.   Refrigerate until ready to serve.

Turkey Chili

Ingredients:

Vegetable cooking spray

1 large onion, chopped

1 T garlic, minced

1 ½ lb ground turkey

2 cups water

1 28-oz can canned crushed tomatoes

1 16-oz can canned kidney beans, drained and rinsed

2 T chili powder

2 t turmeric

1 t smoked paprika

1 t dried oregano

1 t ground cumin

1 t hot sauce

Directions:

1.   Spray a large soup pot with cooking spray.

2.   Cook onions until tender and starting to brown.

3.   Add garlic and cook for 30 seconds.

4.   Add turkey and stir frequently until it's fully cooked.

5.   Add water and all the remaining ingredients and bring to a boil.

6.   Reduce heat and simmer, uncovered, for 30 to 45 minutes.

Gingerbread Oatmeal

Ingredients:

1 cup water

½ cup old fashioned oats

1/3 cup dried, unsweetened cherries or cranberries

1 t ground ginger

½ t ground cinnamon

¼ t ground nutmeg

1 T flaxseed

1 T molasses

Directions:

1.   Combine the first 6 ingredients in a small saucepan over medium-high heat.

2.   Bring mixture to a boil. Reduce heat and simmer for 5 minutes or until all of the water has been absorbed.

3.   Add flaxseed, cover and let stand for 5 minutes.

4.   Serve drizzled with molasses.

Roasted Chicken Wraps

Ingredients:

½ cup reduced-fat mayonnaise

2 T pickle juice

1 t freshly cracked black pepper

1 ½ cup shredded red cabbage

1 T apple cider vinegar

¼ t kosher salt

¼ t cayenne pepper

1 deli-roasted chicken, cooled

6 whole wheat or mixed grained flatbread

Directions:

1.   Combine mayonnaise, pickle juice and pepper in a large bowl and refrigerate.

2.   In a medium bowl, add cabbage, vinegar, salt and cayenne pepper. Toss to mix.

3.   Remove and discard skin and bones from chicken and shred into bite-sized pieces.

4.   Add chicken to mayonnaise mixture and stir to thoroughly combine.

5.   Divide chicken and cabbage mixtures evenly between the flatbread slices and roll to secure.

Brazil Nut-Crusted Tilapia with Sauteed Kale

Ingredients:

¼ cup roasted Brazil nuts

½ cup fresh bread crumbs

2 T grated Parmesan cheese

¼ cup whole grain mustard

1 ½ lbs tilapia fillets

vegetable cooking spray

1 T sesame oil

1 clove garlic, mashed

1 ½ head kale, chopped

¼ t kosher salt

2 T toasted sesame seeds

Directions:

1.   Preheat oven to 400 degrees F. Lightly grease a baking sheet and set aside.

2.   Place Brazil nuts in a food processor and pulse until finely ground. Transfer to a small bowl and stir in breadcrumbs and Parmesan cheese.

3.   Place tilapia fillets on a baking sheet and spread evenly with mustard.

4.   Divide Brazil nut mixture evenly over tilapia and lightly spray breadcrumbs with cooking spray.

5.   Bake for 8 to 10 minutes or until tilapia is cooked through.

6.   Meanwhile, heat a large cast-iron or stainless steel skillet over medium-high heat.

7.   Add sesame oil and heat for 15 seconds, then add garlic.

8.   Cook for 20 seconds then add the chopped kale.

9.   Cook while stirring frequently until kale is tender.

10.   Add sesame seeds and toss to combine.

11.   Serve fish immediately with a side of kale.

Persimmon and Pear Salad

Ingredients:

1 t whole grain mustard

2 T fresh lemon juice

3 T extra virgin olive oil

1 shallot, minced

1 t minced garlic

1 ripe persimmon, sliced

1 ripe red pear, sliced

½ cup chopped pecans, toasted

6 cups baby spinach

Directions:

1.   In a large bowl, whisk together the first five ingredients.

2.   Add the persimmon and the remaining ingredients and toss well to coat.

Red Pepper and Turkey Pasta

Ingredients:

3 large red bell peppers

3 T extra virgin olive oil

1 large onion, chopped

2 t minced garlic

2 t fresh oregano, chopped

1 T red wine vinegar

2 lb ground turkey

2 lbs hot, cooked, rigatoni

Directions:

1.   Cut peppers in half and remove seeds and stem before coarsely chopping them.

2.   In a large Dutch oven, heat oil over medium heat.

3.   Add peppers and onions and cook for 20 minutes or until very tender.

4.   Add garlic and cook for additional 5 minutes.

5.   Transfer mixture to a blender or food processor and puree until smooth.

6.   Return sauce to pan and reheat over medium-low heat.

7.   Stir in oregano and vinegar and adjust seasonings.

8.   Meanwhile, sauté ground turkey in a large skillet sprayed with vegetable cooking spray. Cook until it starts to brown.

9.   Add browned turkey to the sauce and simmer for 20 minutes.

10.   Serve over hot, cooked pasta.

Roasted Sweet Potato Soup

Ingredients:

2 ½ lbs sweet potatoes

1 T extra virgin olive oil

¼ t kosher salt

½ t freshly cracked pepper

1 ½ cups thinly sliced leeks or onions

1 1-in piece ginger, peeled and minced

1 t minced garlic

½ cup dry white wine

1 t chopped fresh thyme leaves

5 cups vegetable broth

2 cups orange juice

Directions:

1.   Preheat oven to 400 degrees F.

2.   Peel and cut sweet potatoes into 1-in pieces.

3.   Place on baking sheet and toss with olive oil, salt, and pepper.

4.   Place in oven and roast for 45 to 50 minutes until tender and well-browned.

5.   In a Dutch oven or large soup pot that's sprayed with cooking spray, cook leeks over medium high heat until wilted and tender.

6.   Stir in garlic and cook for 1 minute.

7.   Add wine and bring to a boil. Cook until wine has evaporated. Add broth.

8.   Stir in sweet potatoes and thyme and bring to a boil.

9.   Reduce heat and simmer for 20 minutes or until all the vegetables are tender.

10.   Carefully puree soup in batches or use an immersion blender.

11.   Reheat soup before serving.

Steamed Salmon with Lemon Scented Zucchini

Ingredients:

1 onion, thinly sliced

1 lemon, thinly sliced

2 small zucchini, thinly sliced

1 cup white wine

½ cup water

4 6-oz salmon fillets

¼ t kosher salt

¼ t freshly ground pepper

Directions:

1.   Place onion and the next 4 ingredients in the bottom of a large Dutch oven.

2.   Season fish evenly with salt and pepper.

3.   Fit a lightly greased steamer rack over the vegetables in the Dutch oven.

4.   Place over medium-high heat until liquid starts to boil.

5.   Reduce heat to medium-low and carefully place fish on rack.

6.   Cover and steam until cooked through, about 8 to 10 minutes.

7.   Serve fish on top of vegetables and poaching liquid and top with sliced olives. Garnish, if desired.

Chapter 10: An Overview Of Arthritis

It has to be noted that arthritis is not a single disease; it is instead a term used to refer to all rheumatic conditions which total to over a hundred types. The most common types are osteoarthritis, gout, rheumatoid arthritis, and fibromyalgia.

Arthritis involves inflammation of the joints, surrounding tissues, and other connective tissues, and may affect one joint, but there are cases when it affects multiple joints.

This condition may also be present in people with existing conditions like heart disease, diabetes, high blood pressure, and obesity.

The pain that comes with arthritis married with the symptoms of other health conditions is enough to reduce a person's quality of life and to make disease management even more difficult.

However, this is not to say that arthritis is unmanageable. With enough understanding of this ailment, a patient may be able to find ways to ease its symptoms.

Causes

There is no known single cause for arthritis; it varies according to type. As mentioned earlier, there are hundreds of different kinds of this condition, and that means there could be similarly hundreds of causes. Gout, for instance, is a result of an increase in the level of uric acid in the body, while those like fibromyalgia have completely unidentifiable origins.

Symptoms

The term "arthritis" is almost always equated to pain, which is its most common symptom. Severity of pain could vary. It could also be on and off, or chronic. Location of pain would depend on the affected joint.

Stiffness is yet another sign of this condition, and it happens mostly in the morning or upon waking up at any time of the day. This is a result of not moving for long periods; thus, it could also be felt after sitting for hours.

Morning stiffness, however, should not last for more than an hour – so if it does, do inform your doctor.

Swelling is another common symptom, and this is not something to miss because the skin around the affected joint would turn reddish and would feel warm.

Note that if your swelling lasts for three days or longer, or recurs more than three times a month, then you must inform your physician.

Remember that getting out of bed or up from a chair should not be that difficult, so if it does become challenging, start observing your body for other symptoms. Try to keep a record of the time the symptoms appear and the severity. This will help your physician in making a proper diagnosis.

Risk factors

Age is the most common risk factor of arthritis. In fact, people 60 years old and older are most affected by this condition. However, cases of younger arthritic patients have been recorded; there is even one so-called Juvenile Idiopathic Arthritis that affects children and teenagers.

Meanwhile, there are other risk factors to consider.

Gender

There have been studies showing that there are higher cases of arthritis in women, and the CDC notes that about 60% of osteoarthritic patients are females.

Women, compared to men, have more elastic tendons in their lower bodies, and these are what allows the body to endure the enlargement of the stomach during pregnancy. However, the constant movements of these tendons, especially during childbirth, add pressure to the joints, thus making women more susceptible to arthritis.

Moreover, unlike men who have aligned hips and knees, women have hips wider than their knees; thus, they are more prone to injuries, and consequently, to arthritis.

Genes

This is another risk factor of arthritis, and women are said to have a significant genetic link present; in fact, if a mother was diagnosed of osteoarthritis in particular, her daughter will likely develop the same condition at about the same age she incurred it.

This does not mean that men with a family history of arthritis are free from this said risk.

Hormone

Meanwhile, the levels of estrogen, a hormone that originates from the ovaries and protects cartilages from inflammation, decline as women age. This is why women, upon menopause, are at higher risk of developing arthritis.

Uric acid level

Men are more prone to gout because they have higher levels of uric acid than women do. However, after menopause, females start to become susceptible to gout.

Obesity

Extra weight adds pressure to the joints, causing cartilages to wear away more rapidly; it also causes pressure on blood vessels, making joint movement difficult and thereby causing stiffness and sometimes, inflammation.

Nature of work

The most neglected, yet most common, risk factor to note is a person's nature of work. Those who are exposed to repetitive squatting or knee bending are prone to osteoarthritis of the knee.

Lack of movement

It is partial to say that only highly physical work triggers arthritis. A sedentary lifestyle could also lead to this condition since the joints could become stiff due to lack of movement.

Other risk factors

Injuries leave traces of damage that increase susceptibility to pain and swelling, meaning the injured is inclined to develop arthritis. Infection and aut0-immune disorders, meanwhile, are also significant considerations.

Reasons for pain

As said earlier, the joint is covered by cartilages, which are vital because they act as a shock absorber while allowing the joints to move smoothly. When this protection erodes over time, as it does in degenerative arthritis (or if attacked by antibodies, as in inflammatory arthritis), then bone will rub into bone, and the friction this movement creates causes pain, stiffness, and swelling.

Since often, it is not only one joint that is affected by degeneration or inflammation, then pain could be even worse.

Joint degeneration and joint inflammation are what happens when arthritis takes place.

Joint degeneration

The joint is covered by cartilages which serve as its protection and allow its smooth movements. Cartilages are tough and elastic tissues.

Joint degeneration happens when the cartilage starts to wear away. It is, therefore, common in old people whose cartilages have corroded over time.

Joint degeneration is the common cause for osteoarthritis.

Joint inflammation

This takes place in a body that suffers from an autoimmune disorder, in which antibodies attack tissue linings of the joints, causing cartilages to deteriorate. Rheumatoid arthritis is the most common inflammatory arthritis.

Further studies about the roots of each type of arthritis are being conducted continuously to help patients better understand their conditions.

Effects on life

According to AF, "23 million of those suffering from arthritis have limited capability to carry out the most common activities, including both standing and walking."

Arthritis could have different effects on people, but one thing is for sure, the pain that comes with it is troublesome.

Arthritis and work

Pain that lasts for days is enough for a person to frequently file a sick leave, and symptoms that last for months could already influence the decision to resign.

According to AF, more arthritic patients take a break from work compared to those who take leaves due to other medical conditions. Meanwhile, those with osteoarthritis and rheumatoid arthritis miss a combined 172 million workdays every year.

Arthritic patients are often caught between needing to work to sustain medical costs and having to stop because of intolerable symptoms.

Arthritis and depression

With the limitations imposed by arthritic symptoms, patients begin to feel helpless. Thus, despite this condition being physical in nature, its psychological effects are evident: arthritic patients are prone to depression.

About 40% of people with arthritis have been found to suffer from depression as recorded by AF. Unfortunately, this only worsens the symptoms of arthritis since people with such mental condition tend to be inactive and to have poor food intake. These could cause more damage to the cartilage and could lead to further stiffness in the joints.

Arthritis and family

Arthritis may also have significant impacts on families. The luckier patients would enjoy care and understanding from their loved ones, but some breadwinners diagnosed with this ailment were left by their families. On top of all these, the economic impact of arthritis is undeniable. In fact, AF notes that people with such condition "give up potential income due to injury or illness." The financial burden that this condition entails is enough for some family members to give up.

Arthritis and suicide

Sadly, there have been accounts of arthritic patients developing suicidal thoughts. Meanwhile, according to the Medical Journal of Rheumatology, those who actually committed the act did so in a more violent manner compared to others with no said condition who did the same.

Common Types of Arthritis

The list of arthritic conditions could go on and on, but here are some of the types worth noting either for being common, like osteoarthritis, or for being rare, like JIA.

Osteoarthritis

This is the most common type of arthritis and according to the Osteoarthritis Research Society International, it is the result of the body's failed attempt to repair tissues, and it may occur as part of the aging process.

In this condition, the cartilage breaks down, leaving joints rigid, thereby limiting range of movement as stiffness, inflammation, and pain arise.

This condition is usually found in the knees, hips, and hands, and deformity of said joints, if affected, would be visible.

Rheumatoid Arthritis

This condition is categorized as a systematic inflammatory disease, but no definite cause has been identified. There's belief of it being a result of immune system malfunction because there have been findings, though inconclusive, that it occurs when the immune system attacks the soft tissue that produces a fluid to ease joint movement and to nourish the cartilage.

People with rheumatoid arthritis may experience tenderness and pain in the joint area in its early stages. Though over time, they may see redness and swelling. It is also said to affect multiple joints at one time, and may involve other parts of the body, such as nerves, eyes, lungs, and heart.

Symptoms could develop gradually, but there have been accounts of people suddenly becoming unable to get out of bed.

At the onset, people diagnosed of this condition would likely feel unwell and often exhausted; there is constant low fever and poor appetite.

Fibromyalgia

Fibromyalgia has a variety of symptoms affecting different parts of the body. Some of the most common symptoms are muscle and skeletal pain, fatigue, sleep disturbances, mood changes, concentration problems, headaches, and abdominal pain.

Although scientists think that injury, infection, or trauma may affect the nervous system's response to pain, thus resulting in fibromyalgia, there are other claims that it could be due to hormonal changes brought about by a flu virus. It is even suspected to be psychological in nature. As a consequence of its strange origin, this condition is difficult to diagnose.

Gout

Most people with gout experience intense pain and swelling in the big toe, more often following an infection or injury. Consecutive pain may occur on and off in other joints, but mostly in the feet and knee. This pain eventually becomes constant.

Gout is the result of hyperuricemia, a condition in the body that produces excess uric acid. However, obesity and constant alcohol consumption also contribute to the cause of hyperuricemia and gout.

This condition is an inflammatory arthritis that is also linked to increased risks of heart disease, high blood pressure, and kidney stones.

Psoriatic Arthritis

This condition, like fibromyalgia, is said to be difficult to diagnose because it shares symptoms with other forms of arthritis. The most common are painful and swollen joints, sausage-like fingers or toes, tendon or ligament pain, skin rashes, nail changes, fatigue, reduced ranged of motion, eye problems, and flares.

Psoriatic arthritis occurs when the immune system attacks healthy cells in the joints, causing inflammation and overproduction of skin cells. It is most common in people with psoriasis, and it takes place along with other types of arthritis.

Spondyloarthritis

There are two main symptoms for spondyloarthritis: lower back pain, and swelling in the arms and legs.

Scientists have found as many as 30 genes that lead to this condition; however, other causes are unclear. Scientists believe it may be related to some bacteria entering through the damaged bowels.

Reactive Arthritis

The symptoms for this type of arthritis would be inflammation of joints, eyes, bladder, and urethra. Sometimes mouth sores and skin rashes may appear.

Exposure to certain bacteria has been linked to reactive arthritis. The most commonly associated bacteria are Chlamydia Trachomatis, Salmonella, Shigella, Yersinia and Campylobacter.

Infectious Arthritis

Intense swelling and pain, usually in a single joint, is the most typical symptom of infectious arthritis. In half of all cases, infectious arthritis also involves the knee, hips, ankles, and wrists.

Some types of infectious arthritis are caused by bacteria. Though, in most cases, it occurs when an infection somewhere in the body travels through the bloodstream onto the joints.

Juvenile Idiopathic Arthritis (JIA)

The condition is prevalent in children and teenagers, which is why it is called juvenile. The cause of the condition is not known which is the reason it is classified as an idiopathic condition.

Because JIA is believed to be a component of different diseases, no one test can be used to determine its diagnosis. Before symptoms can be classified to be caused by JIA and other medical conditions need to be first ruled out.

This condition are reported to be one in 1,000 children.

Chapter 11: Dealing With Chronic Pain

Chronic pain can last for up to six months and can cripple the person. It can be stressful not just physically but also mentally and those who suffer from it have been shown to be easily irritable due to the frustration.

There are a variety of prescription pain relievers available over the counter that can be used to alleviate the pain of chronic illness, however, as the long-term use of these medications may cause more harm to the body, sufferers are advised to make adjustments in their lifestyle and eating habits in addition to other.

Affecting both emotional and mental health is vital because suffering can lead to depression, which then causes more pain. It can become an endless cycle.

There have been scientifically proven methods of dealing with discomfort. However, patience is when using these methods as the results don't happen over night.

Distraction

It is believed to be a successful method to reduce pain since the mind has been proven to be unable to focus to focus on multiple things at the same time. Therefore, pursuing a pastime which requires concentration can help with discomfort.

Some of these activities include cross-stitching, scale model writing, painting, and cross-stitching. Video games and singing are also recommended. Anything that requires your mind to be focused is beneficial.

Relaxation of the muscles

The tightness of muscles can result in stiffness, which makes it more difficult to move joints. While massages are an effective method of relaxing muscles, it is not recommended for all arthritis sufferers, as incorrect strokes can cause more discomfort. If you choose to get massage, it's recommended to consult an expert. Massages, stretching, and warm baths are however, excellent for easing muscle tension.

Reduce stress

Stress is a natural element of life since it's the body's reaction to tension and pressure.

However, excessive amounts of it can cause the pain, and therefore is particularly harmful for arthritis sufferers who are frequently anxious due to the issues caused by their illness: costs of medical treatment, the inability to function, the side consequences of medication and fears of the future. The ability to handle stress is certainly, essential.

The most common signs and symptoms of stress are muscle tension, anxiety and fatigue, insomnia, and a loss of appetite.

For managing stress Here are some suggestions for managing stress:

1. Identify stressors.

2. Modify what is changeable Accept that which can't be altered.

3. Contact someone for assistance.

4. Accept responsibility for your emotions and do your best.

5. Let your tears flow if you want; it's okay.

6. Make life simpler and eliminate from unnecessary tasks and obligations.

7. Manage your time and energy effectively.

8. Set goals and keep your eyes on them.

9. Laugh.

10. Sleep.

When you are doing all of this be sure to breathe deeply.

Meditation can be a method to relieve stress, however mastery over it can require some time. The relief isn't always easy using this method, but when done regularly and through constant practice, it can be effective in calming the mind and an effort to relax the body. It also aids in achieving a good sleeping, which is crucial in managing pain.

Exercise

Many people suffering from arthritis are anxious about doing exercise, as they worry they will be in more discomfort. However, those suffering from this health issues actually have to exercise, however they should not do it in a vigorous manner. Slow and steady stretches are preferred and should be performed frequently.

Tai Chi is an ancient Chinese martial art which mixes slow, gentle movements and deeply breathing. It is just one of the numerous exercises recommended for arthritis patients. But, it must be practiced under the supervision of experienced instructors. Do not attempt this on your own!

It is beneficial to stretch every day; it aids in restoring range of motion, which is affected by arthritis.

Acupuncture

It is a traditional Chinese technique of treatment that's been practiced over the centuries and that western society has been adopting for a long period of time. It involves needles that are put through the skin to reach specific points of acupuncture. In accordance with the requirements the needles are inserted into various levels.

Acupuncture points are located along meridians that carry Chi energy flows. There are approximately 350 points within the human body. each one corresponds to particular organ or body part. It is important to note that the needle isn't placed in the region of an organ that is affected or body part, but rather in the exact location of the organ's point or points. There are a variety of points that can be used for certain types of diseases.

The concept is to balance the chi within the body since an imbalanced energy can cause diseases. Acupuncture has been proven to be efficient in relieving arthritis patients of discomfort.

Herbal Medicines

Herbalism is a method of healing which makes use of the plant's parts or extracts to treat ailments. It is also a practice that has been practiced for centuries and is a part of all cultures.

The plant medicines are able to be consumed by mouth or applied topically and also those that have anti-inflammatory properties are suggested to arthritis patients in place of NSAIDs due to the lower risk of adverse effects If they do have any.

146

Chapter 12: Nature-Based Medications For

Arthritis

There is a belief that there isn't a cure for arthritis but symptoms may be reduced. Therefore, arthritis sufferers are prescribed NSAIDs in order to deal with the signs of their illness. Similar is the case of herbal remedies which have anti-inflammatory properties are only used to alleviate discomfort.

But, given that arthritis is not curable and is a life-long condition, it could become an ongoing issue. This is why taking NSAIDs even if symptoms are present can be risky since these medications have been proven to cause negative side consequences. This is why herbal remedies gain traction since there aren't any harmful unwanted side adverse effects.

However, this doesn't mean to say that all patients are all likely to react positively to herbal medicines. Since every body is different, there is a chance that each person will react differently to specific plants. This is why taking remedies with herbs is best done with the guidance and supervision by a qualified expert.

Natural Anti-Inflammatories

To the delight of many The truth is that natural painkillers are not difficult to come across Some are available at the table.

In addition, among the numerous kinds of herbal remedies there are some that stand out because of their anti-inflammatory properties. Here are a few the herbs that proved to be beneficial to patients suffering from arthritis.

Aloe Vera

It is a common herb, and is renowned for treating minor abrasions and sunburn. Additionally there are reports of this herb reducing the pain of arthritis patients.

The leaves contain gel-like substances inside, which can be applied topically on painful areas.

Although there are a few people who use aloe vera tea form however, experts don't recommend it for everyone since this plant could cause diarrhea in certain patients. The application of the topical gel has no negative effects, and is usually recommended.

Green Tea

It is a well-loved drink that is well-known because of its anti-inflammatory qualities. Active ingredient Epigallocatechin Gallate (EGCG) is a potent catechin that blocks producing certain inflammation chemical substances in the body.

Green Tea is said to be taken orally in the form of tablets, tea, or tincture.

Ginger

The flavoring that is commonly used in the kitchen is an effective painkiller that is the same as ibuprofen but without the negative impact. Gingerol is the most common chemical that gives ginger its distinctive flavor, is also responsible for the herb's anti-inflammatory effects. Ginger has been shown to decrease certain immune cells, which are normally linked to inflammation.

It can be consumed as tea or as a tincture. It is possible to incorporate it into foods as a flavoring ingredient and can be stir-fried or pickled. However, for those who aren't a fan of the spicy flavor of ginger there are capsules to buy in the form of an over-the-counter (OTC).

Ginger is also utilized as a liniment or compress.

Turmeric

This herb isn't only an extremely popular curry base. It's also the most frequently used painkiller used by arthritis patients. Curcumin, the active component responsible for the dark-colored color in this herbal remedy, is found to possess antibacterial and anti-inflammatory properties which aid arthritic patients in coping with discomfort.

Boswellia can be consumed as tea or tincture. It is additionally available OTC in tablets and creams for topical use.

Cat's claw

Cat's claw originates originated from a tropical plant and has been utilized since the time of the Inca civilization. It's typically utilized to strengthen the immune system. However, research has shown that it is powerful in reducing pain and swelling. However, excessive consumption of this herb may increase the amount of stimulation to the immune system and , consequently, worsen the pain of arthritis. Therefore, it is recommended to consult the advice of a doctor.

The herb is able to be consumed in tincture or tea, however there are tablet versions OTC.

Rosehip/ Rose hip

This plant is the rose's fruit It is the thing left after every single flower of the rose have been sucked away. It's rich in vitamin C and also contains polyphenols and anthocyanins. These are believed to help reduce joint inflammation and damage through reducing the production of inflammation enzymes and proteins. As a result it is recommended to patients suffering from arthritis.

Rosehip can be consumed as a raw drink or used in tinctures or teas. You can also buy OTC capsules that contain it as well.

Other natural supplements

It is crucial to supplement your diet to ensure that our body is functioning correctly. Here are a few supplements that can aid in the treatment of arthritis and they are all OTC.

Fish Oil

Omega-3 Omega-3 of fish oils blocks cytokines as well as prostaglandins, and transforms them into powerful anti-inflammatory compounds called resolutionins.

Anti-inflammatory treatments can be prepared.

To reap the benefits from the use of herbs, it's essential to prepare them properly. Here are some guidelines for making teas, liniments, or tinctures. There are various methods of making herbal preparations, but they are most likely to work best with the herbs mentioned in this section.

Teas (fresh herbs)

* If using roots remove the skin first, and then cut into smaller pieces. If you are using leaves, there is cutting is not necessary.

* Place the the herb in a pot and let it sit for a while in water.

* Bring to the boil and simmer for 30 minutes.

* Strain.

* Mix in honey or stevia to lessen the strong flavor.

* Drink cold or warm.

Teas (dried herbs)

* If you're using dried roots, cut them into smaller pieces. If not move on to the next step.

* Wrap the herbs in cheesecloth.

* Put the herb in a pan and let it steep in water.

* Bring to the boil and simmer for 30 minutes.

* Strain.

* Mix in honey or stevia to lessen the strong flavor.

* Drink cold or hot.

Liniments

This is intended for use by the public!

Choose a herb: it can be fresh or dry.

* Put a 1 ounce of this herb in an container.

* If using dried herb, add five tablespoons of rubbing alcohol in the jar. If it is fresh, use just two pounds.

The bottle should be sealed and let it sit for 2 weeks. Be sure to shake it regularly.

* Strain into clean bottles

* Note: Label appropriately to prevent accidental consumption.

Rub the affected areas whenever you feel it is necessary.

Tinctures

They are thought as more powerful than tea however, they have alcohol in them. This is why it's recommended only as a preventative measure to treat arthritis and not as a treatment option for those already suffering from the disease. Alcohol can interact with other medications.

* Place 4 ounces of dried herbs into a jar.

* * Add another 20oz 100 proof vodka.

Cover the jar with a seal and store the jar in a cold and dark location for at least two weeks.

* During the two weeks, be sure that you shake the jar every day.

Once you are ready then strain through cheesecloth, squeeze the herbs out.

* It is possible to refrigerate it.

* It is possible to ingest it in its pure form or diluted with water or juice.

Hot compresses of herb

* Blend the herb until it is coarse.

* Wrap in cheesecloth.

* Steam it over boiling water, or put it in boiling water.

* Remove the herb that has been heated.

* Wrap your body in a warm, soft cloth.

* Press the area that is painful.

Chapter 13: Stretches To Treat Arthritis

Contrary to popular perception that arthritis patients must be confined to a chair in order to avoid stress, they must move and stretch in order to prevent aggravating their pain.

Inactivity creates stiffness in ligaments and muscles, making it harder for joints to move. This also hinders the burning calories, leading to weight gain which increases the risk of developing arthritis.

But this doesn't mean that arthritis patients are unable to take on any kind of exercise they wish. They just need to stretch to reduce stiffness and maintain their joints' flexibility.

While stretching it, your range of motion restored. This is the range that joints are capable of reaching, and people with arthritis are limited by this.

Here are a few stretching exercises which can help arthritis patients. Keep in mind that the 'hold' listed in the list will take between 5 and 10 seconds. You can increase it to 20 seconds,

157

however, only if you feel that it won't strain your body instead.

Neck stretch

• Bring the right ear up to your right shoulder, and gently hold, then let it go.

Then slowly bring your chin towards your chest and then keep it there until you are able to let it go.

• Bring the left side of your ear up to your shoulder, and hold it; then let go.

Shoulder Stretch

* Shake shoulders at least a couple of times.

* Reach towards the sky, reaching as high as you can.

* Sit straight or sit.

* Keep your arms to your body.

* Arms open at the shoulder height.

* Bend elbows.

* Keep your palms facing forward.

* Pull shoulder blades towards each other.

* Move arms up and over.

Keep elbows to keep them in line with the body.

* Put arms down.

* Shake shoulders.

Arm Stretch

* Sit straight or sit.

* Place your arms by your sides.

* Bend elbows.

* Turn thumbs to the back towards shoulders.

* Lift one arm up overhead and reach for the shoulder opposite.

* Use the opposite hand to keep the elbow of your bent arm in place.

* Do the same thing for your other hand.

Shoulder and Wrist The Stretch

* Place fingers and palms together.

* Spread your arms out in the direction of your body by keeping fingers and palms together.

* Pull your hands towards your chest.

* Extend your elbows upwards.

* Bring your palms together as you move it closer to your body, squeeze your shoulder blades into the process.

Finger Walk Stretch

* Sit down with your hands on the table.

* Point your fingers forward.

* Move your thumbs towards each one.

* Move the fingers of your hands one at a toward the thumb.

* Hold your hands up.

* Reposition it to its original position on top of the table.

Hands and Wrists Stretch

• Gently turn your wrists while moving your hands around in a circular motion.

* Fist for just a few seconds.

* Spread your fingers wide and large.

* Stand in front of the wall.

* Rotate your arms upside down.

Press your palms on the wall.

* Lift your hands up towards the wall gradually.

Calf and Hip Stretch

* Keep your posture straight.

• Keep your abdominal muscles in a good shape.

* Spread your arms and hands the wall

* Straighten your elbows.

Spread your feet to the extent of your hip.

Keep your hips and shoulders a straight position.

* Put one foot behind the other leg.

* Bend the knee of your front foot while keeping your heel on the back foot on the floor.

* Hold.

* Repeat for the next leg.

Knee Bend

* extend one leg.

* Bend knee 90 degrees.

* Bring knee closer to arms.

* Hold.

• Release, repeat the same leg.

Knee Stretch

* Sit in a straight line on the chair.

* Raise one knee to the highest you can (do not bend your back).

* Lower your foot to the floor gradually.

Leg as well as Ankle Stretch

* Sit straight and straight.

* Slowly straighten your knee.

* Flex one leg slightly.

* Point your toes straight ahead.

* Point your toes towards the ceiling.

* Lower your leg.

* Repeat for the second leg.

Ankle Stretch

* Sit straight.

* Extend your legs and put them in front of you.

* Slowly turn feet to one side.

* Repeat the process in the opposite direction.

Calves that stretch

* Keep two feet from an unfinished wall.

* Rest both hands against the wall.

* Lean towards the wall.

Make sure your feet are level on your floor.

Maintain your spine straight.

* Hold the position.

Repeat the release and repetition.

Stretching Hamstrings

Spread your body flat across the back.

* Make a knee bend.

* Pull your thigh up.

* Bring your thigh up towards your chest.

* Stay in your position.

Repeat the process on your second leg.

Heel/Toe Stretch

* Sit in a straight line on the chair.

Place your feet flat on the floor.

* Take your heels off and hold (make sure to keep your feet in place).

* Return to the flat position to your feet.

* Lift your feet and hold them for a few seconds.

Walking

* Walk every day.

Make sure you maintain a good posture when walking.

Always begin with gentle stretching then, as your body is accustomed to moving, the difficulty level may be increased, if you wish. Be sure to stretch every day.

Chapter 14: Prevention Measures

There has been debates about what is most important which is the best time to treat arthritis or what to manage it. Some provide early treatments using drugs such as Adalimumab (Humira) to prevent the condition from becoming worse.

It is true that the best prevention remedy for arthritis is to lower the risk of it, or delaying time of onset. Therefore, it is important to keep joints in good condition as long as you can.

To achieve this, some modifications in diet, lifestyle and routines are needed.

Foods to Avoid

Although studies on the relationship between food and arthritis prevention remain unconclusive, experts recommend arthritis patients to avoid certain foods often associated with joint pain.

Trans-fat

This type that is fat was proven to cause joint pain in a number of patients. It is found in dairy and beef products however in a small amount. However, it is abundant in processed or manufactured food items.

Make sure you drink plenty of water to flush out the salt.

Sugar

Reduced sugar intake is essential not just for arthritis patients however, it is for all of us because it is a source of calories that our bodies may not be able to fully burn. Sugar is the cause of obesity and weight gain that can trigger joint discomforts.

It's not just only limited to table sugar. certain types of carbohydrates transform into sugar when they are inside the body. So, cutting down on foods that are high in this ingredient can help lower blood sugar levels as well.

If you find that food and drinks are tasteless and bland, you can try using the sweetener stevia instead. It is an South American shrub and is naturally sweet. The leaves can be used to

167

sweeten However, recently, powdered versions have been made available.

Alcohol

Although experts have discovered that alcohol can have an anti-inflammatory effect and can actually decrease the risk of developing arthritis it should be noted that this is only the case when it is taken in moderation as well as if person drinking the drink hasn't been diagnosed with arthritis as of yet.

The consumption of alcohol by patients suffering from arthritis is not recommended anymore as it can cause reactions with medicines particularly NSAIDs like naproxen and ibuprofen.

In any event the patient suffering from arthritis uses alternative or herbal medication, moderate consumption of alcohol (a glass a day) could be acceptable. But, experts suggest because alcohol can be addictive and addictive, a complete stop is the best option.

Habits to change

The activities we engage in every day could cause arthritis. Therefore, it is essential to make some changes in our lifestyle.

Weight gain is a result of a diet.

It is said time and time again that weight gain is a major risk factor for arthritis as it places greater stress on joints, which causes cartilages to be worn away more quickly. Therefore, changing your diet could greatly help.

Get more fiber in your diet in your diet by taking more of a whole grains and fruit and vegetables However, do not try to make major changes in your food habits because this could cause you to allow yourself to be enticed by your cravings and then lose the weight and much more. Start small and take small steps.

Uncomfortable shoes

The shoes can stress the muscles of the legs, which can cause stress to joints. It's time to put down your uncomfortable shoes, particularly the stilettos. Choose shoes that feel comfortable and help your feet relax.

Lifestyle of sedentary

Most people nowadays are glued in front of their TV or computer screens. What they aren't aware of is that staying in a sedentary position hurts their bodies, as it causes stiffness in joints and muscles, making it difficult to move. Make sure to stand up for some time and stretch.

Chapter 15: Whom To Talk To About Arthritis?

If you suspect you're showing signs of arthritis, consult your physician. Perform a physical exam to determine if you're suffering from arthritis. Your doctor will let you know whether an Rheumatologist or arthritis expert needs to be consult. In the meantime, if you suffer from arthritis and surgery is needed, an orthopedic surgeon might be consulted.

When the arthritis affects different body parts, specific specialists such as dermatologists, ophthalmologists or dentists, could also be part of medical teams according to the part of the body that is affected.

If you're thinking of using alternative therapies such as herbal medicine, it is important to inform your doctor first about your choice. Look for an herbalist who is certified. This person is highly trained in herbal medicine and will ensure that you're using herbs in the correct way. Be aware that even though herbal remedies are readily accessible, it's recommended to use it under the supervision and guidance of a qualified doctor.

Other experts to talk to regarding alternative treatment options for arthritis include a holistic physician licensed or certified acupuncturist, an ayurvedic health sciences doctor or oriental medicine doctor or a diplomatic Chinese herbologist or a naturopathic doctor.

Keep in mind that for everything that is health-related seeking advice from a professional is necessary. Do not self-medicate as it could cause further harm in your body.

Chapter 16: Conventional Rheumatoid Arthritis

Treatment

If you visit a doctor for joint pain, it is important to be prepared for your visit. Be prepared to answer any questions and describe your symptoms will assist the doctor to provide the right treatment for you. Here are some tips you can try to do to get the most benefit from your doctor's appointment.

Prior to the Visit

Before you go to the doctor you must make an inventory of the following:

* All your symptomsmust be described and include as much detail as you can.

* Your medical background

* Any supplements or medications that you currently take

* Questions you may have for your doctor

During Your First Visit

Your doctor might ask you questions that will help him or determine the cause of your problem and suggest possible treatment options. The questions could revolve around symptoms duration, the joints affected, changes in the symptoms, which actions cause symptoms to become worse when, what time of the day does your pain the worst or how your symptoms impact your daily activities. As well as asking questions and looking over your joints, your doctor might suggest a couple of tests, including blood tests or X-rays. It's crucial to realize that RA might not be identified through tests if it's found earlier because the condition isn't long enough to have lasting changes to the body. Based on the information gathered during the visit, your physician can recommend a range of treatments.

Traditional Treatment Alternatives

Although there isn't a cure for RA but there are some traditional treatment options that can ease the pain, reduce the inflammation, and stop further damage that is caused by RA. In general, the method of treatment will depend on the extent of your RA. If it's detected earlier, a less invasive treatment strategy could be recommended. If you're RA is from moderate to severe treatments tend to be more intensive. If you're RA is severe, treatment options could include the most intense treatments. A comprehensive treatment plan that takes your quality of life into account could comprise medications, occupational or physical therapy educational and counseling, exercise routines or diet therapy, as well as surgery. Remember every treatment plan must be tailored to your particular situation. Because there isn't a cure, the goal of treatment is to achieve remission.

Medication

There are two primary purposes of the drugs that are prescribed to treat RA. The first type of medication is prescribed to ease the symptoms. The other kind of medicine is prescribed to stop the damage due to RA and stop the decline in joint health.

Pain Relief

If you're able to take regular non-prescription pain relief like Acetaminophen or acetaminophen.

However, these medications not be sufficient because they do not decrease inflammation. Instead, you should use anti-inflammatory medications. Most of the time, your doctor may suggest a nonsteroidal anti-inflammatory medicine (NSAID) like naproxen sodium or ketoprofen. They are available either in OTC or prescription forms. If you decide to use an OTC or prescription is contingent upon the degree of inflammation and discomfort. The doctor may suggest the lowest dose of an NSAID that is mild NSAID at first. If the dose isn't adequate to treat your condition, the doctor may raise the dosage. If this doesn't work then the doctor may suggest trying another NSAID. They can be administered by mouth or via a cream which is applied to the skin of your painful joints. It's crucial to realize that NSAIDs can only treat manifestations of RA and are not effective in stopping the progression that causes the condition.

Halting the Activity of Disease

While NSAIDs typically work in moderate cases, if your RA is getting worse the doctor might suggest taking the disease-modifying antirheumatic drug (DMARDs). DMARDs help reduce inflammation, as well as reducing joint damage. In most cases, DMARDs work by suppressing the immune system, which helps to lessen the negative effects of RA. The most commonly used DMARDs are methotrexate leflunomide, or sulfasalzine. Certain doctors might prescribe a mix of DMARDs. They are taken orally, or injected or via IV. Because DMARDs require at minimum two weeks to start functioning, your doctor might suggest the use of an NSAID in order for you use for a while.

The Side Effects

Like all medications that is prescribed, the medications that are used to treat RA can cause negative side adverse effects. A few of the potential adverse side effects range from mild to more serious. For instance, NSAIDs may cause upset stomachs and fluid retention as well as damage to kidneys or the liver. DMARDs may cause the sensitivity of sunlight, nausea, diarrhea mouth sores, loss of hair or birth problems, liver damage and suppressing bone marrow. Along with these adverse consequences, biologics weaken the immune system, which can expose you to infections. In addition, corticosteroids can cause the retention of fluids, mood swings and mood swings, diabetes, osteoporosis and increased risk of getting infections. If your doctor recommends using medication as a treatment option to treat your RA be sure to discuss the potential side consequences with your physician.

Physical Therapy and Occupational Therapy

If your RA is getting worse to the point of affecting your daily activities Your doctor might suggest that you undergo physical or occupational therapy to help you regain flexibility for your joints. Physical therapy is a form of exercise that helps help restore dexterity to your joints. Apart from exercising, a physical therapy therapist might use massaging, ice, or heat therapy to aid joints stay flexible. In terms of occupational therapy, this kind of therapy can help you understand how to live your life in spite of having RA. A therapist in occupational therapy can assist you find easier methods of completing routine tasks that take your RA into account. A therapist in occupational therapy may suggest assistive devices that will aid you with the routine tasks that can be difficult because of the RA. For instance there are levers you can attach to doorknobs. It's much easier for those suffering from RA to pull an object than to turn the knob. The aim of both physical and occupational therapy is to improve the quality of your life to ensure that you are able to function at or near the level you used to prior to RA with minor adjustments.

Surgery

If your RA is very severe or medical treatments haven't stopped the progression your joints could develop deformities, which can cause limitations in motion and severe discomfort. If your RA is so severe it can be a major negative effect on your life quality. If you're suffering from this the doctor might suggest surgery. In the course of the procedure, the damaged joint is removed and a replacement joint is inserted. The replacement joints are usually constructed from plastic or metal. The replacement joint will allow you to return to your standard of life. If the injury to your joint has led to tendon injury, surgery could be needed to fix the tendon. In the event that joint replacement is not feasible due to your specific case of joint injury it is possible to have the joint joined to ensure that the joint can be repaired and used. If surgery is recommended you consult with your doctor regarding the possibility of success and the chance of complications following surgical procedures on your joints.

Find Help as Early as Possible and ensure it's Round

The methods mentioned above are the core of the conventional treatment for RA. It's best to tackle RA head-on and as early as possible. Beginning treatments at the time of the beginning of RA as is possible, minimizes the risk of joint injury. This also provides quicker relief from the discomfort that RA can cause. Get medical attention if you start to experience symptoms. Discuss with your doctor about the options available for you. It is important to inquire with your doctor about all the options for treatment available. Find a comprehensive treatment program that is multi-faceted and specific to your needs.

Conclusion

I hope that this book is capable of providing you with valuable information in controlling you Rheumatoid Arthritis manifestations. Although RA can be a crippling illness, making the right food choices can aid in battling it and reduce the discomfort.

It is now time to adhere to the tips I've given those in the book, and don't allow Rheumatoid arthritis to control your life. I wish you the best as you attempt to conquer and manage the rheumatoid arthritis.

www.ingramcontent.com/pod-product-compliance
Lightning Source LLC
Chambersburg PA
CBHW060335030426
42336CB00011B/1345